Integrating Acceptance and Commitment Therapy with Islāmic Psychotherapy for Managing Chronic Pain

This book proposes a psychotherapeutic intervention integrating Islāmic Psychology with Acceptance Commitment Therapy (ACT) for Muslims with chronic pain conditions.

The first part of the book provides an overview of the challenges of living with chronic pain and illness and explores the cultural expressions of pain and disease and a literature review on culturally adapted psychotherapies. An overview of the main components of ACT and their congruence with Islāmic tenets, including spirituality and contemplation, is provided to propose an Islāmic based ACT approach that aims not to reduce or eliminate pain but rather to help the client build a repertoire of behaviours that lead them towards value-based directions. The second part of the book outlines a session-by-session cultural adaptation of the six core processes of ACT interwoven with Islāmic teachings from the Quran and Sunnah. The book is supplemented with downloadable resources such as worksheets and handouts that professionals can use in practice.

This book is intended as a pain management guide for therapists familiar with ACT and Islām. It will provide therapists with the tools to deliver a faith-adapted, evidence-based treatment for clients who follow the Islāmic faith.

Dr Razia Bhatti-Ali is a Consultant Clinical Psychologist in the United Kingdom. She has been employed in a pain management role for over six years providing clinical interventions, supervision, and support for a psychology team. In collaboration with her Urdu-speaking colleagues, she successfully developed an ACT-based Urdu Pain Management Programme for Muslim service users and also created a digital Urdu version to increase access to the intervention. The outcome data from this initiative were presented at the British Pain Society conference in 2019 and the International Association of Islāmic Psychology conference in conjunction with Riphah University, Lahore. The work has also been published as a book chapter and in two peer-reviewed journals.

Focus Series on Islāmic Psychology

Series Editor: Professor Dr. G. Hussein Rassool

Professor of Islāmic Psychology

About the Series

In contemporary times, there is increasing focus on the need to adapt approaches of psychology, counselling psychology and psychotherapy to accommodate the integration of spirituality and psychology. With the increasing focus on the need to meet the wholistic needs of Muslims, there was a call to adapt approaches to the understanding of behaviour and experiences from an Islāmic epistemological and ontological worldview.

The aim of the Focus Series on Islāmic psychology and psychotherapy is to introduce a range of educational, clinical and research interventions relating to Islāmic psychology and psychotherapy that are authentic, practical, concise, and based on cutting-edge research. Each volume focuses on a particular aspect of Islāmic psychology and psychotherapy, its application with a specific client group, a particular methodology or approach, or a critical analysis of existing and emergent theoretical and historical ideas.

Each book in the Focus Series is written, in accessible language, with the assumption that the readers have no prior knowledge of Islāmic psychology and psychotherapy.

Advancing Islāmic Psychology Education: Knowledge Integration, Model, and Application (2023)
By G. Hussein Rassool

Integrated Research Methodologies in Islāmic Psychology (2024)
By G. Hussein Rassool

Integrating Acceptance and Commitment Therapy with Islāmic Psychotherapy for Managing Chronic Pain (2024)
By Razia Bhatti-Ali

Integrating Acceptance and Commitment Therapy with Islāmic Psychotherapy for Managing Chronic Pain

Dr Razia Bhatti-Ali

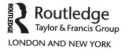

Routledge
Taylor & Francis Group

LONDON AND NEW YORK

First published 2024
by Routledge
4 Park Square, Milton Park, Abingdon, Oxon OX14 4RN

and by Routledge
605 Third Avenue, New York, NY 10158

Routledge is an imprint of the Taylor & Francis Group, an informa business

British Library Cataloguing-in-Publication Data
A catalogue record for this book is available from the British Library

ISBN: 978-1-032-35977-9 (hbk)
ISBN: 978-1-032-35976-2 (pbk)
ISBN: 978-1-003-32962-6 (ebk)

DOI: 10.4324/9781003329626

Typeset in Times New Roman
by Apex CoVantage, LLC

Access the Support Material: https://www.routledge.com/9781032359779

This book is dedicated to Sanah, Aneeqah, and Hana. I pray my work is an inspiration for you. May you always be blessed and guided by the Almighty to live a life of prosperity and piety.

"Seek knowledge from the Cradle to the Grave."

Prophet Muhammad ﷺ

Contents

Illustrations

Figures

Worksheets

Handouts

Preface

This book is a humble attempt to integrate Islāmic principles in the delivery of an Acceptance Commitment Therapy (ACT)-based clinical intervention to meet the challenges of living with chronic pain. The aim is to help Muslims with pain and illness learn to live with their condition while remaining aligned with their Islāmic values.

Building on the success of Cognitive Behaviour Therapy (CBT) as a therapeutic modality for pain management, ACT is one of the third-wave behavioural approaches that have grown as an evidence-based psychological intervention for the management of pain and chronic health conditions. Unlike CBT, the emphasis of ACT is not to reduce or eliminate pain but rather to help the client build a repertoire of behaviours that lead them towards value-based directions that enrich their life and help them to learn to live with chronic pain as best as they can.

ACT proposes that individuals who have psychological or physical difficulties often struggle because they try to reject or avoid their unwanted inner experiences. Psychological flexibility can be cultivated to enable acceptance and committed action to overcome psychological difficulties. The ACT model of psychological flexibility consists of six core processes, which include thought defusion, acceptance, present-moment awareness, values-directed behaviour, committed action, and self as context. Islām is the guiding point to living a values-based life, which is why ACT as a therapeutic modality may be more likely to engage clients from the Muslim community due to its principles being more congenial to an Islāmic approach to life and particularly for those who may find engaging with the collaborative nature of a CBT approach challenging.

From an Islāmic perspective, religious beliefs serve as the compass for living a values-based life. ACT places a strong emphasis on living in alignment with values as a means of enhancing functionality for those individuals who may have lost their sense of purpose in life as a result of their struggle with pain and suffering. ACT suggests that acceptance can help strengthen connections to a variety of long-term values and enable people to live a rich and meaningful existence.

The central ideas of ACT bear some resemblance to Islāmic tenets, such as the virtues of sabr (patience) and shukr (gratitude), which can be applied to help individuals pivot away from fatalistic beliefs and the tendency to externalise health challenges as being beyond their ability to endure. The client is guided towards change by placing focus on long-term consequences through personal experience rather than immediate positive outcomes, such as the avoidance of emotionally distressing circumstances. Islāmic teachings discourage the avoidance of committed actions when faced with challenging circumstances. The Hadith, *"Trust in Allah but also tether your camel,"* reflects the idea that clients should act and engage in self-management rather than take the fatalistic view of relying on God alone to provide a solution.

Islām discourages behavioural excesses and the pursuit of desires for short-term gains and advocates practices that develop a state of being present in the here and now. One such practice is dhikr (remembrance and prayer), which can be used while following a behavioural pattern based on ideals rather than avoiding challenging situations. ACT also advocates the use of present-moment awareness to help create a space in which an individual can learn to step back from the pain and cultivate pain acceptance. This resonates with the Islāmic practice of using prayer and praise of God during difficult times.

The purpose of this book is to offer guidance on delivering an Islāmically integrated psychotherapy incorporating ACT, an evidence-based treatment for managing chronic pain interweaved with Islāmic teachings from the Quran and Sunnah to awaken the client's spirituality and divine connection. The aim to help the pain suffered accomplish spiritual tranquillity while developing acceptance and a commitment to pursue a life based on their core values as Muslims.

Acknowledgements

I begin in the name of Allah, the Merciful and the Compassionate. All praise is due to Allah, from whom we seek help, seek forgiveness, and seek guidance. I would not have accomplished this work or indeed anything else in my life without the grace of Allah Almighty.

I would first like to thank Professor Ghulam Hussein Rassool for offering me the opportunity for this undertaking and for his patience in waiting for the work to be submitted. I would especially like to thank Rehana Hussain, who has offered her unwavering support and guidance throughout this journey. I am truly grateful to her for making time from her busy life to provide constructive assistance. I would like to acknowledge my colleague Mohammed Shoaib who was the one who inspired me to embark on this journey several years ago with his passion for culturally adapted interventions. His input made it possible for me to advance the knowledge required for this project. I also wish to thank my employers for providing me with the opportunity and support to develop this work and for helping lay the foundations for pursuing this book project.

I am blessed to have a family who continuously encourages me to pursue my goals and has always celebrated my achievements. I thank my amazing parents in their heavenly abode who made me the person I am today and supported all my endeavours throughout their life. I pray Allah gives them the highest of ranks in Jannatul Firdaus.

I would like to thank all the people who, through their unique expertise, have knowingly and unknowingly provided opportunities for me to meet with like-minded people and attend training that has been invaluable in helping me increase my knowledge of Islām to enable this humble work to reach fruition. I pray to Allah for forgiveness for any shortcomings and mistakes I may have made with the contents of this book.

Note to Readers

The book is supplemented with downloadable resources that can be found at www.routledge.com/9781032359779. They feature the worksheets and handouts that appear in the Appendices and are intended for professionals to print and use in practice with clients.

Part 1

1 Introduction

The Challenge of Living with Chronic Pain and Illness

Pain that is experienced for more than three months is known as chronic pain or persistent pain. Chronic pain prevalence rates in the United Kingdom are uncertain, but it is argued that between one-third and one-half of the population is estimated to experience chronic primary pain (Fayaz et al., 2016). Chronic pain is a huge public health problem due to the substantial economic and social burden it creates. It not only affects the individual as a sensory and emotional issue but also impacts the family and social spheres. An appreciable proportion of chronic pain patients experience depression, mood fluctuations, anxiety, altered perceptions and cognition, and emotional instability (Surah et al., 2014).

Living with chronic pain strips people of their ordinary and meaningful elements and the state of existence that we consider "normal." People experiencing chronic pain and illness are frequently forced to slow down due to undesired bodily and emotional symptoms leading to complexities related to loss and grief and impaired physical functionality, which can directly hinder them from engaging in ordinary everyday activities. Those affected by pain and chronic illnesses often get caught up in a vicious cycle a viscious cycle of pain and reduced activity and report considerable challenges with self-management and psychological distress leading to poor quality of life (Hadi et al., 2019).

The average person endures chronic pain with an additional layer of associated emotional distress, which is likely to increase the perception of pain sensations. Figure 1.1 shows how chronic pain causes secondary complications, which subsequently increases the perception of pain.

Vidyamala Burch in her book Living Well with Pain and Illness explores the Buddhist saying: *"Pain is inevitable, suffering is optional."* She describes how the Buddha compared chronic pain to being struck by two arrows. The individual who does not resist physical pain feels the initial arrow, but their journey with chronic pain, after an initial experience of grief and a sense of loss, may result in lasting transformation and existential advantage. For others, the agony of the associated psychological distress is akin to being shot with a second arrow which

DOI:10.4324/9781003329626-2

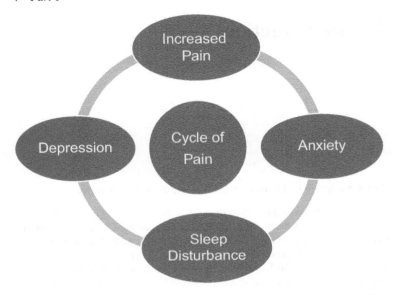

Figure 1.1 Vicious Cycle of Pain and Distress

is the suffering caused by the mind. These individuals are also more likely to experience a grief reaction and often look for a quick fix to overcome the pain, which may present as withdrawal from life and enjoyed activities.

The parable *"In life, we cannot always control the first arrow. However, the second arrow comes from the possibility of choice"* suggests that we can choose to react to our difficulties even when we cannot change them. The second arrow which refers to our emotional and psychological response to adversities is a natural response but often creates more suffering by limiting and cluttering our minds and preventing us from seeing clearly the appropriate path of action.

Just as patients with diabetes expect a long-term plan involving nutrition, exercise, medicine, education, and prevention rather than control after a single course of treatment, those living with chronic pain also require a holistic approach. Setting realistic expectations and a long-term strategy to manage pain with full awareness of the complexity of the problem is essential to avoid unnecessary stress for the people we treat. This involves recognising the limitations of painkillers and the dangers of prolonged use of non-steroidal anti-inflammatories and opioid analgesics. The latter is linked to a well-publicised "opioid crisis" with rising addiction rates and overdose (Jalali et al., 2020).

Primary care clinicians have a pivotal role in initiating and developing long-term pain management strategies that are multidimensional and integrative and consider the patient's biological, psychological, social, and spiritual needs. Chronic pain management aims not to eliminate the pain but to adjust its threshold to become bearable and help reduce disability and distress by integrating physical, psychological, spiritual, and practical techniques to improve quality of life.

Cultural Expressions of Pain and Illness

It is well documented that, though pain is a personal experience, societal, cultural, and psychological factors affect how people respond to pain (Lipton & Marbach, 1984). However, pain is not just a physical sensation but also has an emotional component that can trigger responses that significantly impact how the pain is manifested, the social context in which it occurs, and the associated pain behaviour.

The biopsychosocial framework helps us understand how the development and maintenance of chronic pain are affected by different factors, but it can also be argued that other less explicit processes impacting pain perception are culture, religion, and spirituality. Every social and cultural group has its vocabulary for expressing pain and anguish (Vance, 2004). Culture strongly determines how it is communicated and the response to it by others. While some cultural groups encourage stoicism, restraint, and downplaying the pain, others demand an excessive display of emotion when faced with suffering (Bhatti-Ali & Shoaib, 2019).

Studies of religion and mental health identify "Positive religious coping" as a spiritual practice that facilitates healing and resilience in the face of adversity (Mir et al., 2015). Positive religious coping refers to people taking a proactive approach to deal with problems by engaging in religious beliefs and practices without solely relying on divine intervention. On the contrary, those who engage in "negative religious coping," hold the notion that God has abandoned them or that the affliction is a punishment. This style of coping has been found to increase psychological distress and pain severity for people with physical illnesses (Ano & Vasconcelles, 2005).

Medical experts struggle to understand the expression of pain in people from cultures other than their own. For some people, it may not be just culture that influences their expression of pain but also religious beliefs (Vance, 2004). A study on back pain in Australian aborigines found that, when compared with the local Caucasian population, the aborigines with back pain did not seek medical treatment or complain because their pain was not perceived as a health problem (Zborowski, 1952). Another study found that Hispanics experience more pain from their health issues than their Caucasian counterparts, especially during depressive episodes (Hernandez & Sachs-Ericsson, 2006).

Cultural representations of pain, spirituality, and religious beliefs may impact health and wellness and attitudes towards life and death (Dedeli & Kaptan, 2013). During illness, spiritual beliefs are more likely to come to the forefront with an increased willingness to use religion to facilitate understanding and acceptance. Faith may empower or comfort people during pain and help them live more meaningful lives (Mir et al., 2019).

For Muslims, living with chronic pain can be an opportunity to ponder and reflect on their lives and reconnect with their spiritual traditions and their divine disposition (fitrah) which is to become closer to God. This helps catalyse the soul's growth, enabling the formation of virtues and character centred on existential fulfilment and wisdom. We know from the work of John Bowlby (Bowlby, 1958) that having a stable attachment has been related to overall wellness, coping and resilience, and healthier relationships. While Spiritual interventions may be culturally, and religiously variable, Prayer is a universal spiritual practice that has the power to produce a feeling of attachment to an unseen power. For Muslims, a healthy attachment to God is likely to be linked to better mental health. "*And whosoever puts his trust in Allah, then He will suffice him*" (Quran, 65:3).

Barriers to Engaging in Therapeutic Interventions

The Muslim population in Western nations has advanced rapidly. Yet, most Western practitioners have little understanding of Islāmic principles and teachings to incorporate within their treatment modalities. For Muslims, Islām is a way of life, a set of moral principles, social norms, and ethical principles that can aid in their ability to tolerate stress and create effective coping mechanisms.

A key barrier to effective pain management interventions is a lack of understanding of the beliefs of patients and their families. The obstacles to inclusive healthcare for Muslims experiencing physical and psychological distress stem from stereotypical perceptions and a health system unprepared to provide linguistic and culturally appropriate care. Healthcare providers are often unaware of their prejudices and assumptions which lead to a negative influence on pain evaluation and misperception of patients from diverse cultural backgrounds (Bhatti-Ali & Shoaib, 2019).

The establishment of pain management programmes based on the biopsychosocial model is an evidence-based and cost-effective effort to help patients with chronic pain regain function and enhance their quality of life (BPS, 2019). Despite the successful outcomes reported, there is a poor uptake of such services with low treatment outcomes for Muslim patients, which may reflect the failure of these programmes to acknowledge the interplay of culture, spirituality, and religiosity in the development and maintenance of psychological effects in those with chronic pain conditions. If the interventions are inconsistent with recognising how beliefs and values affect individuals, this may deter Muslim patients from participating in standard treatment programmes (Lipton and Marbach, 1984).

The majority of public health literature on health disparities emphasises ethnicity more than religion. Given that Islām is a way of life, for many Muslims, faith identity may be more important than ethnic identity, regardless of an individual's level of religiosity. Additionally, research has demonstrated that religious identity is a significant factor that affects well-being and recovery (Koenig et al., 2012). People from different ethnic groups may share common cultural characteristics stemming from generations; however, a faith identity binds cultures together and provides a foundation for core values and principles, hence the importance of focussing on religious identity, values, and principles.

Muslims often take a fatalistic view of their difficulties and may attribute pain, illness, suffering, and injury to Allah's will or due to punishment for their wrongs, especially when a psychological element is involved. These beliefs may function as a barrier to seeking help for their condition. Healthcare practitioners familiar with the Islāmic faith are likely to be more successful in delivering care in a culturally sensitive manner. Health disparities in the treatment of physical and psychological health can be effectively addressed by introducing faith-based interventions.

Therapeutic interventions that reflect cultural beliefs and religious practices by using teachings from the Quran and Sunnah can encourage self-management whilst also preserving faith in divine help. For instance, maintaining physical health and honouring the body are encouraged in the Quran and Hadith as it benefits emotional, psychological, and, most importantly, spiritual existence.

Potential language barriers can be addressed by providing information that is not just literally translated but also conceptually sound. Furthermore, it is not uncommon for health services to use interpreters who speak a different dialect to the patient. It is crucial to ensure that dialectical differences are tailored to the patient's needs when using interpreting services, as otherwise linguistic nuances can be misunderstood and misinterpreted.

Islāmic Perspective on Pain and Illness

Pain and illness have a way of interfering with a person's natural disposition (fitrah), but by examining the emotional roadblocks triggered by pain, people can realign themselves with their values and evaluate their spiritual state. The material world, according to Islām, is characterised by strife because trials and tribulations help people restore their true selves and enable a realisation of their full potential through the struggle with their nafs (ego/self). *"And it may be that you dislike a thing which is good for you and that you like a thing which is bad for you. Allah knows but you do not know"* (Quran 2:216).

The importance of emotions and the necessity of controlling them through faith and reason are both acknowledged in the Quran. For instance, fear is a strong emotion that can be psychologically unhealthy, but if controlled and properly aligned with the fear of divine justice, it can be a fear that is beneficial to one's spiritual development. Therefore, for Muslim patients, being in a place of pain can raise the nafs and give them spiritual freedom and meaning.

As Victor Frankl (2004) said, the primary motivation for human beings is to search for meaning when faced with difficult and painful situations. This view resonates with the Islāmic concept of pain and loss. Islām considers the material world a temporary abode with trials and tribulations that enable the afflicted person to realign with their true selves (fitrah) and grow spiritually. Suffering is thus beneficial and an expected and necessary component of the human condition and can be overcome with trust in Allah. *"And whosoever is conscious of Allah, He will make for them a way out"* (Quran 65:2).

An essential part of the journey of a person with chronic pain, both as a patient and as a person, is the search for meaning which can lead to the possibility of inner growth and spiritual reawakening. Furthermore, chronic pain from an Islāmic perspective provides an objective meaning based on the recognition that life's circumstances are beyond our control and that there is a divinely predetermined good in all outcomes.

This view is exemplified further by the following Quranic verses: *"We burden not any person, but that which he can bear"* (Quran 6:152) and *"Allah charges a soul only with that which is within its capacity"* (Quran 2:286). These verses can inspire people who struggle to deal with life's challenges to use prayer to cultivate a state of well-being. Uncontrolled emotions are inevitable, but learning to sit with them fosters spiritual growth and protects mental health.

Allah tests people to create a new direction and motivates people to change; *"God is with those who are patient in adversity"* (Quran 2:153). Sometimes, it takes a catastrophic situation to help us change. Trials and tribulations have been sent down by Allah to every Prophet and messenger to provide ordinary people with positive lessons for our lives. Prophet Ayyub (AS), also known as the Prophet Job, is famous for his extraordinary patience in facing Allah's trials. Some important lessons can be derived from his life which can help inspire those living with chronic pain and illness.

One of those lessons is to be grateful and submissive in good and bad times. Prophet Ayyub (AS) was tested by Allah with his wealth, family, and his health, for years. Despite this, Ayyub (AS) did not falter in his submission and remained grateful to the Almighty as he endured with patience despite his losses. His story has been honoured in the Quran: *"And (remember the story of) Job, when he prayed to his Lord- (My Lord), indeed, I have been afflicted with sickness, whereas You are the Most Merciful Lord of all the Merciful"* (Quran 21:83).

Ayyub (AS) continued to practice patience and fortitude until Allah(swt) answered his prayer after eighteen years. His suffering is an example of living life with sincerity regardless of the weight of the trial and the number of losses as he realised that all property and descendants did not belong to him but were entrusted to him by God which could at any time be taken back by Him.

And We will surely test you with something of fear and hunger and a loss of wealth and lives and fruits, but give good tidings to the patient, who, when disaster strikes them, say- Surely, we belong to Allah and verily to Him do we return. Those are the ones upon whom are blessings from their Lord and mercy. And it is those who are the [rightly] guided.

(Quran 2:155–157)

Allah tests us to correct us, direct us, protect us, and perfect us. When faced with afflictions, we realise what our priorities are and can correct the path we are travelling on. A problem in life can be a blessing in disguise because it can avert a more undesirable situation that we would have faced and if not in this life, we are promised a reward in the afterlife for our trials. The Quran tells us *"And be patient, for indeed, God does not allow the rewards of those who do good to go to waste"* (Quran 11:115).

The cactus plant is referred to as Sabbar and derives its name from the Arabic word Sabr which means patience. The analogy of the cactus plant aptly describes sabr. Rather than passively waiting for environmental conditions to change or rain to fall from the sky, the cactus pushes its roots deep into the soil and resolutely reaches for those invisible underground streams to store water for difficult days and perseveres with endurance.

The Quran states *"So be patient with gracious, beautiful patience"* (Quran 70:5). Patience or sabr does not imply that we accept suffering or deny our emotions or advocate indifference to emotions by remaining passive. On the contrary, sabr is the trust in Allah's plan to wait patiently for what He decrees, knowing it will ultimately be worth it. Sabr is the struggle for our ideals with gratitude. By practising sabr, we concede that although our pain and emotions are unpleasant, we can find comfort and healing in their darker aspects. Sabr is an active engagement with life while embracing our struggles with tenacity and perseverance.

Therefore, in Islām, the trials of life are a test from Allah and an opportunity for self-improvement to foster the development of qualities such as being patient, forgiving, and grateful. *"Do the people think that they will be left to say, "We believe" and they will not be tried?"* (Quran 29:2). This verse highlights the need for Muslims to accept hardships as part of Allah's power, goodness, and justice and find comfort in the belief that trials and tribulations enable emotional and spiritual transformation. Physical or mental suffering is thus an integral part of the human experience.

When dealing with poor physical or mental health, we often conflate the situation making living with the challenges of pain more difficult. With enduring conditions such as chronic pain, rather than struggling to eliminate or avoid suffering, we must change our relationship with it. A person with chronic pain may strengthen their sense of responsibility by believing that everything happens for a reason and that though they cannot control everything that happens to them they can choose ways of responding. Thus, acceptance can help people achieve inner healing, even if they know they must live with chronic pain. It can also help them become more present and willing to live a life aligned with their values.

References

Ano, G. G., & Vasconcelles, E. B. (2005). Religious coping and psychological adjustment to stress: A meta-analysis. *Journal of Clinical Psychology, 61*(4), 461–480. https://doi. org/10.1002/jclp.20049

Bhatti-Ali, R., Shoaib, M., & Hussain, R. (2019). Delivering a culturally adapted pain management programme: A pilot study presented at the British pain society. *ASM, 2019.*

Bowlby, J. (1958). The nature of the child's tie to his mother. *International Journal of Psychoanalysis, 39,* 350–371.

Burch, V. (2008). *Living well with pain and illness.* Piatkus Books.

Dedeli, O., & Kaptan, G. (2013). Spirituality and religion in pain and pain management. *Health Psychology Research, 1*(3), e29. https://doi.org/10.4081/hpr.2013. e29

Fayaz, A., Croft, P., Langford, R. M., Donaldson, L. J., & Jones, G. T. (2016). Prevalence of chronic pain in the UK: A systematic review and meta-analysis of population studies. *BMJ Open.* https://bmjopen.bmj.com

Frankl, V. E. (2004). *Man's search for meaning: The classic tribute to hope from the Holocaust.* Rider.

Hadi, M. A., McHugh, G. A., & Closs, S. J. (2019). Impact of chronic pain on patients' quality of life: A comparative mixed-methods study. *Journal of Patient Experience, 6*(2), 133–141. https://doi.org/10.1177/2374373518786013

Hernandez, A., & Sachs-Ericsson, N. (2006). Ethnic differences in pain reports and the moderating role of depression in a community sample of Hispanic and Caucasian participants with serious health problems. *Psychosomatic Medicine, 68*(1), 121–128. https://doi.org/10.1097/01.psy.0000197673.29650.8e

https://bigthink.com/culture-religion/this-buddhist-parable-can-ease-your-pain-during-a-crisis/

Jalali, M. S., Botticelli, M., Hwang, R. C., Koh, H. K., & McHugh, R. K. (2020). The opioid crisis: A contextual, social-ecological framework. *Health Research Policy and Systems, 18,* 87. https://doi.org/10.1186/s12961-020-00596-8

Lipton, J. A., & Marbach, J. J. (1984). Ethnicity and the pain experience. *Social Science & Medicine, 19*(12), 1279–1298.

Mir, G., Ghani, R., Meer, S., & Hussain, G. (2019). Delivering a culturally adapted therapy for Muslim clients with depression. *The Cognitive Behaviour Therapist, 12,* E26. https://doi.org/10.1017/S1754470X19000059

Mir, G., Kanter, J. W., & Meer, S. (2013). *BA-M treatment manual addressing depression in Muslim communities.* University of Leeds. http://medhealth.leeds.ac.uk/info/615/research/327/addressing_depression_in_muslim_communities

Mir, G., Meer, S., Cottrell, D., McMillan, D., House, A., & Kanter, J. W. (2015). Adapted BA for treatment of depression in Muslims. *Journal of Affective Disorders, 180,* 190–199.

Surah, A., Baranidharan, G., & Morley, S. (2014). Chronic pain and depression. *Continuing Education in Anaesthesia Critical Care & Pain, 14*(2), 85–89. https://doi.org/10.1093/bjaceaccp/mkt046

Vance, L. M. F. (2004). The role of culture in the pain experience. *Surgical Physician Assistant, 10*(9), 29–37.

Zborowski, M. (1952). Cultural components in responses to pain. *Journal of Social Issues, 8*(4), 12–30. https://doi.org/10.1111/j.1540-4560.1952.tb01860.x

2 Literature Review on Cultural Adaptations for Muslim Patients

Overview of the Literature on Culturally Adapted Therapies for Chronic Pain

Existing research on the cultural adaptation of psychotherapy for Muslims primarily focuses on cognitive behavioural therapy (CBT). CBT has a robust evidence base supporting its efficacy in treating psychological and physical health conditions. The NICE guidelines (www.nice.org.uk.) and the American Psychological Association's (APA's) recommendations identify CBT as a first-line treatment for many disorders due to its strong empirical support. As a result, CBT has become the gold standard in psychotherapy.

However, though CBT is effective for Western populations, there is a dearth of evidence to suggest that it has cultural generalisability (Rathod et al., 2013). The application of CBT and its efficacy with different cultures depends on how well the cultural contexts, values, and preferences of the group are integrated into the intervention and the cultural competency and sensitivity of the therapist (Rathod et al., 2010).

To address this concern, several researchers have developed cultural adaptations of CBT for the management of the psychological health of Muslim communities (Naeem et al., 2015; Mir et al., 2015; Meer et al., 2012). Mir and her colleagues adapted a Behavioural Activation intervention for Muslims experiencing symptoms of depression based on "positive religious coping" (Mir et al., 2015). They found encouraging outcomes and highlighted the value of culturally adapted psychological therapies when treating Muslim patients.

Further research exploring the compatibility of CBT with the personal, religious, family, social, and cultural values of Pakistani patients was undertaken by Naeem et al. (2015). The adapted intervention was reported to be more successful than "treatment as usual."

Algahtani et al. (2019) found CBT to be incompatible with individuals from non-Western backgrounds due to cultural variations. Hence, the researchers modified the therapy to incorporate the role of cultural factors. The study raised the importance of developing the appropriate use of language and the translation of psychological concepts for psychological interventions to be

DOI:10.4324/9781003329626-3

effective. The researchers also found that cultural sensitivity led to increased user participation.

A meta-analysis of 16 randomised controlled trials (RCTs) by the Medical Research Council Framework found a statistically significant benefit in favour of culturally adapted psychotherapies (CAPs) for depression when the intervention was for a majority ethnic group in a population rather than a minority group. CAPs were more effective than control treatments (Chowdhary et al., 2014). These studies have highlighted the importance of cultural adaptations of psychological therapies when treating minority groups.

CBT and Third-Wave Therapies and Their Relevance to the Care of Muslims

In terms of chronic pain management, CBT has been an evidence-based psychological treatment strategy for over three decades, with extensive research studies highlighting its effectiveness with chronic pain. (Morley et al., 1999). However, the effectiveness of CBT for chronic pain patients within Muslim communities has not been robustly established and requires further investigation.

A study by Cardosa et al. (2012) examined the effects of a 2-week CBT pain programme in Malaysia, where the cultural adaptation included relaxation techniques accompanied by Islāmic prayer and meditation. The programme encouraged family members to attend at least once during the programme to offer support with self-management yielded good post-programme gains.

Pearce et al. (2015) undertook a religious adaptation of CBT to treat depression in patients with chronic physical health conditions. Patients from the five major world religions (Christianity, Judaism, Islām, Hinduism, and Buddhism) were treated using a manualised approach to help them integrate their religious beliefs, behaviours, and resources within a CBT framework. The strategies taught included contemplative prayer, scripture study, using religious teachings to challenge thoughts, practising gratitude, altruism, and forgiveness, and participating in a religious community.

The results found that the religious adaptation of CBT was not only sensitive to the challenge of being specific for certain religious traditions but was also broad enough to apply to the diversity of beliefs in the different religions. The researchers argued that the emotional well-being of patients who integrated their religious beliefs, behaviours, and resources with CBT skills was more likely to have positive outcomes.

Similarly, Edwards et al. (2016) investigated the relationships between chronic pain and religious faith among older individuals from five distinct faith groups (Christians, Hindus, Sikhs, Jews, and Muslims). The researchers emphasised the importance of understanding faith/belief and how it is expressed in the context of other aspects of their identity when in distress.

It was found that, for all faiths, religious activities such as prayer played a significant role in the self-management of pain and helped maintain a relationship with God while promoting a calming effect and increased coping. The spirituality of Muslim patients was bolstered by the strength they drew from the rituals of their faith, such as prayer and reciting verses from the Quran.

This study concluded that, while there were aspects of the self-management of pain common across faiths, there are also multi-faceted characteristics of the pain experience, which are unique to particular doctrines, including prayer, the meaning of suffering, and karma. Hence, religious, spiritual, and psychological factors are equally important as the physical aspects of pain when considering cultural adaptations of health interventions.

Though CBT has been the core psychological approach for chronic pain, many studies consider Acceptance Commitment Therapy (ACT) a promising innovative approach to managing chronic pain and other incapacitating medical conditions (Feliu Soler, 2018; Lin et al., 2019).

Since the publication of the first ACT study by Zettle and Hayes (1986), over 1000 RCTs and 422 reviews and meta-analyses have been conducted across the globe and show that ACT is as good if not better as a treatment modality for reducing distress and managing psychopathology (Gloster et al., 2020).

A few studies found no significant differences compared with either treatment as usual, CBT, or waiting list controls (Avdagic et al., 2014; Lanza et al., 2014). ACT is effective with a diverse range of clinical conditions, including depression, anxiety, post-traumatic stress disorder, obsessive-compulsive disorder, chronic pain, the stress of terminal illness, workplace stress, anorexia, substance abuse, and even schizophrenia with the majority of the studies focusing on anxiety, pain, depression, and long-term conditions (Ost, 2008; Powers et al., 2009).

There is little research evidence on the use of ACT for Muslim patients experiencing chronic pain conditions. Bhatti-Ali et al. (2019) developed an Islāmic adaptation of a standardised pain management programme using ACT principles which they piloted with a group of service users. The programme included promoting a values-based life through the use of Quranic stories and metaphors from authentic Hadith sources. Self-management, relaxation, and physical activity were promoted to help cultivate psychological flexibility and resilience. The participants made statistically significant improvements in terms of self-efficacy and the management of symptoms of anxiety and depression following the programme (Bhatti-Ali & Shoiab, 2023).

Subjectively, the participants developed a better relationship with their body and persistent pain and reported an increase in motivation to act on their values. The participants responded well to the six core processes of ACT and appreciated the religious content of the sessions. The results from the pilot evaluation indicate a substantial value in delivering an Islāmically adapted ACT intervention for Muslim patients.

With the dearth of research in this area, future research involving a more robust evaluation with larger samples is warranted to shed more light on the effectiveness of using an Islāmically integrated ACT-based approach for managing chronic pain. There is a strong need for an evidence base for such interventions and evaluation data that are relevant and applicable to Muslim communities.

References

Algahtani, H., Almulhim, A., AlNajjar, F., Ali, M., Irfan, M., Ayub, M., & Naeem, F. (2019). Cultural adaptation of cognitive behavioural therapy (CBT) for patients with depression and anxiety in Saudi Arabia and Bahrain: A qualitative study exploring views of patients, carers, and mental health professionals. *The Cognitive Behaviour Therapist, 12*, E44. https://doi.org/10.1017/S1754470X1900028X

Avdagic, E., Morrissey, S. A., & Boschen, M. J. (2014). A randomised controlled trial of acceptance and commitment therapy and cognitive-behaviour therapy for generalised anxiety disorder. *Behaviour Change, 31*(2), 110–130. https://doi.org/10.1017/bec.2014.5

Bhatti-Ali, R., & Shoiab, M. (2023). Culturally adapted pain management services – in British Muslims and health. In S. A. Dogra (Ed.), *British Muslims, ethnicity and health inequalities.* Edinburgh University Press.

Bhatti-Ali, R., Shoiab, M., & Hussain, R. (2019). Delivering a culturally adapted pain management programme: A pilot study BJP ASM poster abstracts 2019. *British Journal of Pain, 13*(2), Supplement 15–47.

Cardosa, M., Osman, Z. J., Nicholas, M., Tonkin, L., Williams, A., Aziz, K. A., Ali, R. M., & Dahari, N. M. (2012). Self-management of chronic pain in Malaysian patients: Effectiveness trial with 1-year follow-up. *Translational Behavioural Medicine, 2*(1), 30–37.

Chowdhary, N., Jotheeswaran, A. T., Nadkarni, A., Hollon, S. D., King, M., Jordans, M. J., Rahman, A., Verdeli, H., Araya, R., & Patel, V. (2014). The methods and outcomes of cultural adaptations of psychological treatments for depressive disorders: A systematic review. *Psychological Medicine, 44*(6), 1131–1146. https://doi.org/10.1017/S0033291713001785

Edwards, R. R., Dworkin, R. H., Sullivan, M. D., Turk, D. C., & Wasan, A. D. (2016). The role of psychosocial processes in the development and maintenance of chronic pain. *The Journal of Pain, 17*(9 Suppl), T70–T92. https://doi.org/10.1016/j.jpain.2016.01.001

Feliu Soler, A., Montesinos, F., Gutiérrez-Martínez, O., Scott, W., McCracken, L., & Luciano, J. (2018). Current status of acceptance and commitment therapy for chronic pain: A narrative review. *Journal of Pain Research, 11*, 2145–2159.

Gloster, A. T., Walder, N., Levin, M. E., Twohig, M. P., & Karekla, M. (2020). The empirical status of acceptance and commitment therapy: A review of meta-analyses. *Journal of Contextual Behavioural Science, 18*, 181–192.

Hann, K. E. J., & McCracken, L. M. (2014). A systematic review of randomized controlled trials of acceptance and commitment therapy for adults with chronic pain: Outcome domains, design quality, and efficacy. *Journal of Contextual Behavioural Science, 3*(4), 217–227. https://doi.org/10.1016/j.jcbs.2014.10.001

Hayes, S. C. (2019). State of the ACT evidence. *Association for Contextual Behavioural Science.*

Hayes, S. C., Strosahl, K., & Wilson, K. (1999). *Acceptance and commitment therapy: An experiential approach to behavior change.* Guildford Publications.

Hughes, L. S., Clark, J., Colclough, J. A., Dale, E., & McMillan, D. (2017). Acceptance and commitment therapy (ACT) for chronic pain: A systematic review and meta-analyses. *The Clinical Journal of Pain, 33*(6), 552–568. https://doi.org/10.1097/AJP.0000000000000425

Lanza, P. V., García, P. F., Lamelas, F. R., & González-Menéndez, A. (2014). Acceptance and commitment therapy versus cognitive behavioural therapy in the treatment of substance use disorder with incarcerated women. *Journal of Clinical Psychology, 70*(7), 644–657. https://doi.org/10.1002/jclp.22060

Lin, J., Scott, W., Carpenter, L., Norton, S., Domhardt, M., Baumeister, H., & McCracken, L. M. (2019). Acceptance and commitment therapy for chronic pain: Protocol of a systematic review and individual participant data meta-analysis. *Systematic Reviews, 8*, 140. https://doi.org/10.1186/s13643-019-1044-2

McCracken, L. M., Vowles, K. E., & Eccleston, C. (2005). Acceptance-based treatment for persons with complex, long-standing chronic pain: A preliminary analysis of treatment outcome in comparison to a waiting phase. *Behaviour Research and Therapy, 43*(10), 1335–1346. https://doi.org/10.1016/j.brat.2004.10.003

Meer, S., G. Mir, A. Serafin. (2012). *Addressing Depression in Muslim Communities,* University of Leeds.

Mir, G., Meer, S., Cottrell, D., McMillan, D., House, A., & Kanter, J. W. (2015). Adapted BA for treatment of depression in Muslims. *Journal of Affective Disorders, 180*, 190–199.

Miyazaki, E. S., Banaco, R. A., Domingos, N. A., Martins, G. B., & Miyazaki, M. C. (2023). Acceptance and commitment therapy for chronic pain: a quasiexperimental study. *Estudos de Psicologia (Campinas). 40*(209).

Morley, S., Eccleston, C., & Williams, A. (1999). Systematic review and meta-analysis of randomised controlled trials of cognitive behaviour therapy and behaviour therapy for chronic pain in adults, excluding headache. *Pain, 80*, 1–13.

Naeem, F., Phiri, P., Munshi, T., Rathod, S., Ayub, M., Gobb, M., & Kingdon, D. (2015). Using cognitive behaviour therapy with South Asian Muslims: Findings from the culturally sensitive CBT project. *International Review of Psychiatry, 27*(3), 233–246.

Ost, G. (2008). Methodological comparison of clinical trials of acceptance and commitment therapy versus cognitive behaviour therapy: Matching apples with oranges? *Behaviour Research and Therapy, 47*(12), 1066–1070. https://doi.org/10.1016/j.brat.2009.07.020

Pearce, M. J., Koenig, H. G., Robins, C. J., Nelson, B., Shaw, S. F., Cohen, H. J., & King, M. B. (2015). Religiously integrated cognitive behavioural therapy: A new method of treatment for major depression in patients with chronic medical illness. *Psychotherapy (Chic), 52*(1), 56–66. https://doi.org/10.1037/a0036448

Powers, M. B., Vörding, M. B. Z. V. S., & Emmelkamp, P. M. (2009). Acceptance and commitment therapy: A meta-analytic review. *Psychotherapy and Psychosomatics, 78*(2), 73–80. https://doi.org/10.1159/000190790

Rathod, S., Phiri, P., Harris, S., Underwood, C., Thagadur, M., Padmanabi, U., & Kingdon, D. (2013). Cognitive behaviour therapy for psychosis can be adapted for minority ethnic groups: A randomised controlled trial. *Schizophrenia Research, 143*(2–3), 319–326. https://doi.org/10.1016/j.schres.2012.11.007

Rathod, S., Phiri, P., Kingdon, D., & Gobbi, M. (2010). Developing culturally sensitive cognitive behaviour therapy for psychosis for ethnic minority patients by exploration and incorporation of service users and health professionals views and opinions. *Behavioural and Cognitive Psychotherapy*, *38*, 511–533.

Zettle, R. D., & Hayes, S. C. (1986). Dysfunctional control by client verbal behavior: The context of reason giving. *The Analysis of Verbal Behavior*, *4*, 30–38. https://doi.org/10.1007/BF03392813

3 Introduction to Acceptance Commitment Therapy (ACT)

What Is ACT and How Can It Help with Chronic Pain?

ACT is one of the third-wave approaches developed by Hayes et al. (1999) and is based on the principles of positivity, context, perspective, spirituality, and multiculturalism. In terms of chronic pain, ACT works to reverse the negative patterns that those living with pain may have developed over the years. Converse to the traditional approaches to pain management, which focus on pain reduction and are based on the idea that "pain is bad" and must be eliminated to live a free and healthy existence. ACT purports the view supported by research from the fields of relational frame theory and functional contextualism that chronic pain is not the enemy that needs to be controlled or eliminated, but, instead, it is the struggle with pain that creates suffering (Hayes, 2004).

Values based living is considered important in ACT as it helps to increase functionality for those individuals who may have lost direction in life due to the struggle of living with a chronic pain condition. Rather than putting life on hold, the meaning of life can be reconsidered by reconnecting with core values and thereby undoing unhelpful behaviours that maintain pain and suffering. In this way, people can persist in engaging in normal meaningful activities despite pain.

The ACT approach seeks to assist individuals in accepting the challenge of suffering rather than postponing their lives to manage it. ACT attempts to help people reverse the unhelpful behaviour patterns that they may have developed in their attempts to avoid pain as they are more likely to be harmful to the body and mind than helpful (Rose et al., 2023).

At the heart of ACT is psychological flexibility which can help those with chronic pain start to accept experiences rather than avoid them due to fear of aggravating pain, choose to live with present-moment awareness rather than being in a state of autopilot, and take the actions required to increase agency rather than being incapacitated by unwanted thoughts, emotions, or

DOI:10.4324/9781003329626-4

sensations. The goal of ACT is not to reduce pain but to help people accept that while pain is undesirable, their lives do not need to be paused (Hann & McCracken, 2014). Attempts to avoid pain can sometimes cause more functional limitation and damage than good by negatively impacting both body and mind. ACT encourages letting go of the struggle and accepting chronic pain instead of avoiding it (Burch, 2008).

Choosing actions consciously in the moment instead of reacting out of habit helps build resilience to the challenges of living with pain. In terms of pain management, the model of psychological flexibility that ACT advocates encourages chronic pain patients to drop the agenda of control and embrace unpleasant experiences as part of life (Harris, 2011). The therapy helps the patient cultivate a willingness to change their previous strategies for control and develop acceptance instead of trying to change thoughts or feelings about pain. Accepting negative emotions such as fear, worry, or irritation rather than fighting them constantly is likely to promote the growth of actions that serve valued goals. Assisting the client to identify personal values and goals that living with pain may have hindered is an important aspect of the pain management journey (Hayes, 2004).

The six core ACT processes are (1) acceptance, which means that progress can only be made if the patient demonstrates a willingness to experience some discomfort while pursuing a goal-directed life; (2) cognitive defusion, which entails patients learning to simply acknowledge thoughts and sensations as they occur and without any judgement; (3) present-moment awareness in which the patient is helped to cultivate being grounded in the present moment and to focus on experiences as they occur in real time rather than allowing their mind to drift into the past or the future; (4) self as context which the patient is helped to shift perspective from becoming entwined with their pain to becoming more self-aware and able to observe their self as separate from their thoughts and sensations; (5) values which is one of the main goals of ACT and aim to help patients who in fear of pain have forsaken valued activities and thus may have experienced mood disorders. Patients are assisted in refocusing their priorities, away from pain and towards valued activities; and (6) committed action is when patients identify goals aligned with their values and make the commitment to pursue them (Hayes, 2012).

Review of the Evidence Base for the Efficacy of ACT in Pain Management

The National Institute for Health and Care Excellence (NICE, 2021) reviewed the efficacy of ACT for chronic pain and stated that the ACT helped improve quality of life and sleep while reducing pain and psychological distress. Numerous studies on ACT for chronic pain show that, even three years after ACT therapy, the participants sustained wide-ranging effects of the intervention, including enhanced physical and social functioning and decreased pain-related medical visits (Vowles & McCracken, 2008; McCracken & Gutiérrez-Martínez, 2011). Increased acceptance of pain was linked to improvements during treatment, including reduced anxiety, depression, and disability (McCracken et al., 2005; Vowles & McCracken, 2008).

McCracken and Vowles measured both acceptance of pain and values-based action in a sample of people living with chronic pain and found that these processes are related to important aspects of functioning over time. At a three-month follow-up, an increase in values-based action was linked to improvements in the same areas (Vowles & McCracken, 2008). The researchers indicated the importance of exploring each of the core processes in the overall model from ACT.

McCracken and Gutiérrez-Martnez's findings supported these results in a later study in which the study sample reported increased pain acceptance, reduced levels of depression, pain-related anxiety, and physical and psychosocial disability during the active phase of treatment and at a three-month follow-up, regardless of changes in pain levels. The participants reported increased values-based action and higher levels of psychological flexibility. Much of the uncontrolled effect sizes were medium or large at follow-up (McCracken & Gutiérrez-Martínez, 2011). Treatment process research has also shown that psychological flexibility is significant in adjustment to chronic pain and disability (Hayes et al., 1999; McCracken & Vowles, 2014).

Further support can be seen in a study by Wicksell et al. (2010), who examined the change processes following an ACT intervention for chronic pain and the effects on life satisfaction and disability and found that ACT significantly improved outcomes for those with chronic pain. In a study comparing post-treatment outcomes of pain patients treated with ACT and CBT, the ACT participants had an increased level of improvements in pain interference, sadness, and pain-related anxiety and higher levels of satisfaction than the CBT participants at four-week and six-month follow-ups (Wetherell et al., 2011).

Hann and McCracken (2014) reviewed several studies looking at primary and secondary outcomes and found that ACT is highly effective in improving physical functioning and lowering distress. However, the researchers advised that future RCTs should explicitly identify outcomes as primary and secondary while measuring process variables and psychological flexibility components.

An updated review by Hughes et al. (2017) found that ACT as an intervention for chronic pain was superior to the controls (waiting list or treatment as usual), with measures of pain acceptance, functioning, anxiety, depression, and psychological flexibility showing significant effects. However, pain reduction and quality of life were not significantly different between the comparison groups.

More recently, a systematic review by Ma et al. (2023) found ACT to be an effective treatment for chronic pain and was comparable if not better than other available treatments. Furthermore, Miyazaki et al. (2023) assessed psychological inflexibility, pain intensity, quality of life, anxiety and depression, self-efficacy, and social support among patients with chronic pain and concluded that ACT is a promising treatment for the interdisciplinary treatment of chronic pain.

ACT and Islām

Yavuz (2016) argues that there are parallels between ACT's model of psychological flexibility and Islām. The six processes described by Hayes (2004) can be used as a useful framework for developing Islāmic-based psychotherapy and may be valuable in increasing cultural and religious sensitivity within the standardised treatments for chronic pain.

Acceptance from an Islāmic perspective can be illustrated with the concept of "sabr," an Arabic word translated as patience, persistence, self-discipline, and perseverance in the face of hardship. Sabr means being able to stand firm rather than passively accepting difficulties. This concept can inspire individuals to strive for a meaningful life by developing acceptance of the affliction instead of struggling with aversive situations. The Quran places importance on patience and perseverance in the face of adversity. *"Seek God (Allah)'s help with patient perseverance and prayer. It is indeed hard, except for those who are humble"* (The Holy Quran 2:45).

> *"Oh, you who believe! Seek help with patient perseverance and prayer, for God is with those who patiently persevere."*
>
> (Quran 2:153)

The view of Sabr is often coupled with the "Shukr" meaning gratitude. A Hadith (narratives based on the teachings of the Prophet ﷺ) narrates that Prophet Muhammed ﷺ, said,

> *How excellent is the case of a faithful servant – there is good for him in everything and this not the case with anyone except him. If prosperity attends him, he expresses shukr (gratitude) to Allah (SWT), and that is good for him. If adversity falls on him, he endures it patiently (with sabr), and that is good for him.*
>
> (Pervez, 2014)

Cognitive defusion enables people to step back from their thoughts, images, and memories by *"making closer contact with verbal events as they really are, not merely as what they say they are"* (Hayes et al., 2012, p. 244). Defusion can be achieved by unravelling from the trap of unhelpful thought content and observing them as just thoughts. A common metaphor for defusion is to view the mind as the sky with thoughts being like passing clouds, transient and not permanent with new thoughts rising into and out of awareness until they disappear. This metaphor resonates with the Quranic verse *"For indeed, with hardship will be ease"* (Quran 94.5) as the thought or state of discomfort is not everlasting.

ACT uses present-moment awareness to tune in to what is happening in the moment to detract from becoming caught up in worry and rumination. Focusing attention on the here and now helps people experience life in real time rather than missing each precious moment. Similarly, from an Islāmic viewpoint, being present in mind helps people to appreciate Allah's moment-by-moment creation and is the path to experiencing the real meaning of life and its true purpose. The Prophet Muhammed ﷺ advised a companion *"Constantly be mindful of Allah, and you will find Him Omnipresent"* (Hadith 19, 40 Nawawi).

The ACT model describes the self as context as self-awareness or the "observing self" which is the part of our self that notices sensations, thoughts, feelings, and the images that pass through the mind. Within the Islāmic faith, the concept of nafs (the self) can be understood in relation to the self and the soul, *"And remember your Rabb inside your-self"* (Quran 7:205). By being present in mind, it is possible to have clarity on the realities of both mental and emotional states without becoming attached to erroneous self-stories or limiting beliefs. In Islām, the act of "tawba" (repentance) is a process of behaviour change devoid of the need to remain attached to self-stories (even if those self-stories are linked to unacceptable past actions). The Holy Quran states *"Indeed, Allah will not change the condition of a people until they change what is in themselves"* (Quran 13:11).

Chronic pain conditions often lead to people chasing short-term and limiting methods of relief and avoidance of values-based activities. In the process, activities such as exercise, socialisation, social relationships, engagement in family and community events, prayer, and spiritual practice are sacrificed. The emphasis of ACT on long-term outcomes rather than immediate beneficial results, such as avoidance of painful circumstances, helps patients embrace and commit to change. Islāmic teachings also discourage the avoidance of committed actions when faced with aversive situations. The Hadith, *"Trust in Allah but also tether your camel,"* demonstrates the idea that patients should act and engage in self-management rather than take the fatalistic view of relying on God alone to provide a solution (Edward-Moad, 2018).

The Islāmic faith highlights the significance of taking decisive action (committed action) even when one is inclined to act towards avoiding pain as a means of achieving spiritual growth. The Holy Quran states: *"Allah does not burden a soul beyond that it can bear"* (Quran, 2:286). *"No misfortune ever befalls except by permission of Allah. And whoever has faith in Allah – he will guide his heart. And Allah is Knowing of all things"* (Quran 64:11).

Within the ACT model, the absence of sadness is not a "normal" state, but instead, pain, difficulties, and unpleasant experiences are inevitable and natural consequences of life pain, difficulty, and unpleasant experiences are unavoidable and are the natural outcomes of the human condition (Hayes et al., 2012). Similarly, Islām recognises that suffering and unpleasant experiences are tests of life that are unavoidably unpredictable. This perspective can encourage people to take responsibility for their psychological and physical well-being while acknowledging that pain and suffering may be a test from the Almighty. *"Indeed, Allah will not change the condition of a people until they change what is in themselves. And when Allah intends for a people ill, there is no repelling it"* (Quran 13:11).

References

Burch, V. (2008). *Living well with pain and illness.* Piatkus Books.

Edward-Moad, O. (2018). *Tying your camel: An Islamic perspective on methodological naturalism.* Yaqeen Institute. https:// yaqeeninstitute.org/omar-

Hadith 19, 40 Hadith an-Nawawi https://sunnah.com/nawawi40:19

Hann, K. E. J., & McCracken, L. M. (2014). A systematic review of randomized controlled trials of acceptance and commitment therapy for adults with chronic pain: Outcome domains, design quality, and efficacy. *Journal of Contextual Behavioral Science, 3*(4), 217–227, ISSN 2212-1447.

Harris, R. (2009). *ACT made simple: An easy-to-read primer.* New Harbinger Publications, Inc.

Harris, R. (2011). *Embracing your demons: An overview of acceptance and commitment therapy.* Psychotherapy.

Hayes, S. C. (2004). Acceptance and commitment therapy and the new behaviour therapies: Mindfulness, acceptance, and relationship. In S. C. Hayes, V. M. Follette & M. Linehan (Eds.), *Mindfulness and acceptance: Expanding the cognitive behavioural tradition* (pp. 1–29). Guilford.

Hayes, S. C., Pistorello, J., & Levin, M. E. (2012). Acceptance and commitment therapy as a unified model of behaviour change. *The Counseling Psychologist, 40*(7), 976–1002.

Hayes, S. C., Strosahl, K. D., & Wilson, K. G. (1999). *Acceptance and commitment therapy: An experiential approach to behavior change.* Guildford Publications.

Hughes, L. S., Clark, J., Colclough, J. A., Dale, E., & McMillan, D. (2017). Acceptance and commitment therapy (ACT) for chronic pain: A systematic review and meta-analyses. *The Clinical Journal of Pain, 33*(6), 552–568. https://doi.org/10.1097/AJP.0000000000000425

Ma, T. W., Yuen, A. S., & Yang, Z. (2023). The efficacy of acceptance and commitment therapy for chronic pain: A systematic review and meta-analysis. *The Clinical Journal of Pain, 39*(3), 147–157. https://doi.org/10.1097/AJP.0000000000001096

McCracken, L. M., & Gutiérrez-Martínez, O. (2011). Processes of change in psychological flexibility in an interdisciplinary group-based treatment for chronic pain based on acceptance and commitment therapy. *Behaviour Research and Therapy, 49*(4), 267–274.

McCracken, L. M., Vowles, K. E., & Eccleston, C. (2005). Acceptance-based treatment for persons with complex, long-standing chronic pain: A preliminary analysis of treatment outcome in comparison to a waiting phase. *Behaviour Research and Therapy, 43*(10), 1335–1346. https://doi.org/10.1016/j.brat.2004.10.003

McCracken, L. M., & Vowles, K. E. (2014). Acceptance and commitment therapy and mindfulness for chronic pain: Model, process, and progress. *American Psychologist, 69*(2), 178–187.

Miyazaki, E. S., Banaco, R. A., Domingos, N. A., Martins, G. B., & Miyazaki, M. C. (2023). Acceptance and commitment therapy for chronic pain: a quasiexperimental study. *Estudos de Psicologia (Campinas), 40*(209).

Pervez, A. (2014, December 30). *Sabr Key to Jannah.* http://messageinternational.org/sabr-is-key-to-jannah/

Rose, M., Graham, C., O'Connell, N., Vari, C., Edwards, V., Taylor, E., McCracken, L. M., Radunovic, A., Rakowicz, W., Norton, S., & Chalder, T. (2023). A randomised controlled trial of acceptance and commitment therapy for improving quality of life in people with muscle diseases. *Psychological Medicine, 53*(8), 3511–3524. https://doi.org/10.1017/S0033291722000083

www.nice.org.uk/guidance/ng193/evidence/f-psychological-therapy-for-chronic-primary-pain-pdf-9071987011

Vowles, K. E., McCracken, L. M., & Eccleston, C. (2008). Patient functioning and catastrophizing in chronic pain: The mediating effects of acceptance. *Health Psychology, 27*(2(Suppl.)), 136–143.

Wicksell, R. K., Ahlqvist, J., Bring, A., Melin, L., Olsson, G. L. (2008). Can exposure and acceptance strategies improve functioning and life satisfaction in people with chronic pain and whiplash-associated disorders (WAD)? A randomized controlled trial. *Cogn Behav Ther. 37*(3), 169–182. doi: 10.1080/16506070802078970. PMID: 18608312.

Yavuz, F. K. (2016). In ACT for Clergy and Pastoral Counselors-Using Acceptance and Commitment Therapy to Bridge Psychological and Spiritual Care Edited by Nieuwsma J, A. Walser R, D. and Hayes S, T. Context Press.

4 Adapting an ACT Intervention for Muslims with Chronic Pain

The Six Processes of ACT

ACT was not developed for any particular diagnosis but, instead, as an application for the human condition to help alleviate suffering. Contrary to the rules of Western psychology, which focus on the notion of healthy normality, ACT therapy acknowledges "abnormality" as a component of the human psyche. For example, happiness is often considered the norm, while unhappiness is considered abnormal leading to a struggle against events that are perceived to cause unhappiness. Yet, this is not always possible, as sometimes the cause of our distress may be related to events that are not within our control.

A prominent example is the COVID-19 pandemic, as a result of which people's rights across the globe were rendered powerless since nothing could be done to alter the situation. Some may have weathered the storm and overcome their psychological distress, while others may have experienced significant physical and mental health issues.

The tools used in ACT can help us build on our strengths to learn how to deal with life and the inevitable adversities that it brings in the knowledge that not everything has an explanation or a solution. Often, the clients entering therapy want the therapist to help remove the problem. However, attempts to prevent or avoid unhappiness and dysfunction by eradicating unwanted experiences may have the paradoxical consequence of increasing pain and a sense of loss of control. The goal of ACT is not to overcome pain or fight emotions but to transform our relationship with complex thoughts, feelings, and sensations and to accept them as transient and harmless, even if uncomfortable. The focus is on transformation via acceptance.

Metaphors are often used in ACT to help illustrate the power of language and how we use relational frames to make sense of a stimulus. One common metaphor used in ACT to describe emotional pain and the futility of trying to control it is the quicksand metaphor. The more we struggle with difficulty, the deeper we sink into the quicksand. However, with less resistance, we have a better chance of becoming unstuck if we roll out of the quicksand instead of struggling.

DOI:10.4324/9781003329626-5

Psychological Flexibility

Psychological flexibility is the capacity to remain in contact with the present moment with full awareness while changing or persisting in behaviour better aligned with values and goals (Biglan et al., 2008; Harris, 2009). In other words, pursuing goals even in the face of adversity. The six fundamental elements for increasing psychological flexibility are cognitive defusion, acceptance, contact with the present moment, values, committed action, and self as context/observing self. An interconnected hexagon traditionally represents the relationship between these processes, called the ACT hexaflex (Hayes, 2005).

The hexaflex is used to work through these six processes to help the client recognise and stop internal event control strategies, observe their experiences in the present moment without judgement or label, and commit to behaviours that elicit flexible and effective outcomes (Hayes, 2005). Each of these six aspects of ACT are used to assist in case formulation and guide treatment. Working through these processes helps to identify the areas of "stuckness" that prevent the individual from living a rich, meaningful life.

Figure 4.1 shows the hexagon representing the six core processes and how these can be used individually or in combination to help cultivate greater psychological flexibility towards a life rich with purpose. These six processes can be divided into three behavioural components: Open (acceptance and defusion), Present (awareness and self as context), and Engaged (values and committed action).

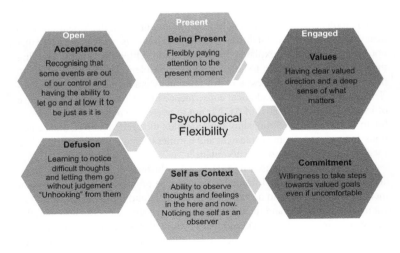

Figure 4.1 Psychological Flexibility

1. *Acceptance*, as opposed to experiential avoidance, can often be misunderstood as passive tolerance or resignation. It can often be unappealing as a concept as many people have preconceived notions that it means "just get over it." However, acceptance refers to the ability to meet our whole experience, even if painful, uncomfortable, or distressing. While it is a natural tendency to avoid discomfort and create strategies to provide short-term relief through experiential avoidance, the problem is that pain is a part of life, and no matter how much we struggle against it, it does not always go away. Harris (2011) refers to unwanted private experiences as "demons" that we must embrace. The struggle and resistance against our "demons" generate needless pain, which eventually turns into extra suffering. Acceptance does not imply enjoying, desiring, choosing, or supporting the circumstance; instead, it is the realisation that some things are beyond our control and letting go of the struggle can allow us to make choices about the things we do have control over such as our actions.

In terms of chronic pain management, acceptance is an integral part of the intervention. Acceptance techniques encourage goal-directed activity, which may involve uncomfortable feelings as the attempt to control emotions is discouraged. Progress can only be made if there is a willingness to experience pain while engaging in activities aligned with values. Rather than trying to escape the pain or its related discomfort, the client learns to see it as normal.

An exercise to build acceptance is to help the client understand that their thoughts and emotions are a natural response to pain and that enjoyable activities do not have to be compromised by the fear of aggravating pain. The cultivation of willingness to focus on emotions and body sensations and to consider what may be holding them back from valued activities is an ingress to the client, realising that they do not have to be controlled by pain or the associated emotional responses. Using metaphors can often help clients understand acceptance better and can be tailored to individual needs. For example, the tug-of-war metaphor illustrates that if we are in a tussle with an opponent that matches our strength, we could be stuck forever, pulling back and forth. The alternative option is to drop the rope and focus our time on something that we can and want to do.

2. *Cognitive defusion* is a skill primarily used to "unhook" or create some distance from our thoughts and emotions and is the opposite of fusion. Fusion occurs when we become entangled with the content of our thoughts, emotions, and experiences. Defusion allows for a radical shift in our context by creating a space between symptoms to help us to recognise thoughts for what they are and not the descriptive "realities" we create. For example, "I am useless" can mean that the individual believes they are useless, and the thought triggers feelings, emotions, and even memories that reinforce this view.

With defusion exercises, people notice their language processes as they expand and observe the thoughts as they come and go as neutral observers without them becoming literal truths that must dictate behaviour. Defusion helps us pause and notice the thought and the reaction that it triggers. With this pause, it is possible to step back from the unhelpful thought and choose not to believe it as a truth. Changing the thought to "I am noticing that my mind is telling me I am useless" or "I am having a thought that I am useless" encourages a greater separation from unhelpful thought content and the space to consider an alternative.

3. *Contact with the present* refers to a non-judgemental awareness of inner and outer experiences in the present moment instead of worrying about the past or future. This means noticing our patterns of life as change can only be made if we are aware of what needs to be changed to help us become more adaptable to change. Simply pausing and noticing what is happening can give us the space to pivot towards what is important. Being present in the moment makes it possible to notice what shows up, even if the current moment is undesirable. It implies that the individual does not reject what is there but instead cultivates a "this is it" attitude towards every moment.

Being aware of the present moment engages various brain centres that temper experiences of pain and can relieve discomfort by regulating the nervous system. It can be practised inwardly and outwardly, formally, and informally. Outwardly, it is having a heightened sense of awareness so that we can pay attention to the cat that ran across the road, the changing colour of the leaves, or the flowers that have suddenly started to bloom even if we were oblivious to them previously. Inwardly, we can begin by noticing feelings and sensations and map them in the body. Simply tapping our fingers against the thumb and becoming aware of the sensory experiences allows us to be grounded in the here and now.

4. *Self as context* is the opposite of self as content. Self as context involves taking the perspective of a situation and exploring objectively how we may be overidentifying with our thoughts, internal scripts, mental images, and emotions and creating limitations in our behaviour. Inversely, self as content is when we become fused and defined by the "I am" labels and includes the existential and deep-rooted beliefs, we hold about ourselves. For example, a person who says "I am depressed" will then develop behavioural rigidity and permit themselves to continue acting depressed or may disengage from others. An antidote to self as content is self-compassion. Perspective-taking is the recognition that we are not the content of our thoughts, emotions, and physical experiences but rather the ones experiencing them.

5. *Values* define what is most important to us and guide our motivation to act on our commitments. People may decide to work on their goals because what they need to do and where they need to go is more important to them than staying in the same place. Russ Harris described values as "*Your heart's deepest desires for how you want to behave, how you want to treat yourself, others, and the world around you; the qualities you want to bring to the things you do*" (Harris, 2019). Values are the qualities that we bring to our actions. For example, if someone's value is to be kind and caring, their actions towards others will be underpinned by kindness.

Values are often mistaken for goals. Goals are the outcomes we aim for, while values reinforce our actions to attain our goals. Buying a comfortable home for the family is a goal, while the value driving this goal is wanting to be caring and supportive. Values inspire and motivate people through life and are analogous to the direction on a compass rather than the destination. A lack of clarity of our values may result in rule-governed or avoidant behaviours that may harm well-being. ACT uses metaphors, experiential exercises, and self-exploration to help people with chronic pain choose or realign with their values.

The bus metaphor often used in ACT illustrates this well. While driving the bus of life, we pick up passengers who represent the unique collection of life experiences, emotions, beliefs, bodily sensations, and instincts. The road symbolises the external aspects of life, the situations, and the people we encounter. Our internal content, including thoughts and feelings, is the unruly passengers travelling in the back of the bus making critical comments that distract the driver from the desired route.

These distracting passengers chip away at resilience by causing distress with a constant bombardment of unhelpful comments and criticisms. Every time we need to go towards something important or change, these unruly passengers enter our awareness. The valuable lessons from this metaphor are that, for optimum health and well-being, it is important to remain focussed on driving the bus in the direction that genuinely matters regardless of the mental noise by using values as the compass that helps steer the bus onto the path towards our goals (Hayes et al., 2004).

Although our experiences are undoubtedly real, it is important to distinguish between objective facts (like the road) and unhelpful thoughts (like a passenger) so that we can act with skill and efficiency towards our goals. This metaphor helps achieve that clarity.

6. *Committed action* is the inverse of control and avoidance. It is engaging in effective actions that align with core values. Committed action is the desire to persevere despite unpleasant internal experiences such as worry, thoughts, emotions, and body sensations. To ensure that committed action is effective, it is essential to be flexible and adaptable to changing circumstances and accept that sometimes there will be failures, but failure is not final. It is easier to take committed action if based on acceptance of the situation, values based, and with clear goals and measurable objectives

Psychological Inflexibility

Several studies have reported that, while psychological inflexibility is malleable, in the absence of intervention, it can become stable over time and has been positively correlated with psychological distress and poor mental health for up to two years prospectively (Hernández-López et al., 2020). From an ACT perspective, psychological suffering is caused by psychological rigidity

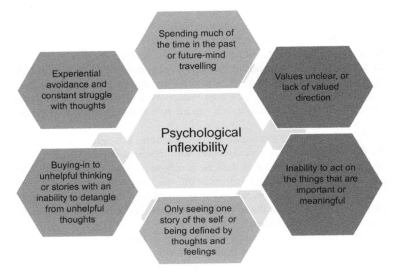

Figure 4.2 Psychological Inflexibility

or inflexibility. The processes that maintain psychological inflexibility and pathology are represented in Figure 4.2.

Psychological inflexibility makes normal functioning and adaptation difficult. It is also one of the aspects of people's life that is likely to cause or exacerbate pain. There are six opposing processes to those described in psychological flexibility. These include a stubborn focus, disregard of our values, inactivity or impulsivity, over-identification with a conceptual self, cognitive fusion, and behaviours characterised by experiential avoidance (Hayes et al., 1996). ACT for pain management facilitates therapeutic progress by guiding the client towards a mindset of psychological flexibility which involves adopting a mindful approach to life and accepting one's situation.

The main principles of the ACT model for chronic pain are that the difficulties that arise when people become stuck in pain and stress are due to the struggle that arises from avoidance and attempts to control, manage, or eradicate pain and the associated discomfort.

Cognitive fusion and fear perpetuate avoidance behaviour. The way people are managing their pain is likely to be creating the chronicity of their difficulties. To live a better quality of life old behaviours may need to be discarded with a willingness to explore new ones. Given the human condition, the ultimate goal of ACT treatment is not to not help the client live without pain and stress but to live well despite feelings of pain and stress. The two ingredients that will enable this transformation are learning acceptance and being willing to move towards value-based goals.

The Junctures Between ACT's Psychological Flexibility Model and Islām

Yavuz et al. (2016) argue that ACT is a congruent intervention to use with Muslim populations communities as their faith and religion are the steering point to living a values-based life and the six processes described by Hayes et al. (2006) that foster psychological flexibility can be used as a useful framework for developing an Islāmic-based intervention and may be valuable in increasing cultural and religious sensitivity within the standardised treatments for those living with physical and psychological challenges. The six processes of ACT and their compatibility with Islām can be examined individually.

Acceptance

Research has shown that avoiding negative thoughts, feelings, and sensations is detrimental to well-being. Instead, having a sense of purpose enables the growth of resilience. Acceptance of painful experiences is the first step towards emotional healing and movement towards a values based life (Hayes, 2004). Acceptance in ACT is founded on the idea that progress can only be made if the person is willing to experience some discomfort while pursuing a life based on what matters to them. The body may be affected by chronic pain, but the decision or capacity to remain true to our values is a choice we can make once we let go of the struggle with physical pain.

The idea of "sabr" in trying times serves as an example of acceptance in the Islāmic faith. Just like ACT does not consider acceptance to be a form of passivity, the Arabic term sabr means showing patience towards any life challenges and facing them with tenacity. Sabr refers to the ability to remain patient, steadfast, and self-disciplined amid difficulties, rather than succumbing to passivity. It involves maintaining one's position and not backing down in the face of adversity. "*So be patient; indeed, the [best] outcome is for the righteous*" (Quran 11:49).

Sabr encourages the individual to strive for a meaningful life regardless of aversive situations. Sabr is the act of having faith and living according to a values based life. Instead of avoiding or struggling with a difficult situation or stimulus, it involves accepting it and letting go of the struggle. The trials of life may seem unending, but having sabr is knowing that the difficulty will end just like a fasting person knows that eventually, the fast will end when the Maghrib call of prayer takes place.

Patience and acceptance in Islām are not simply being immersed in affliction while the world passes by. Life is full of challenges and unfortunately for some more than others. However, during times of despair, the soul can be cleansed by cultivating patience, expressing gratitude, and taking actions aligned with our values.

The Holy Quran makes several references to the connection between being patient and persevering and standing by our values to attain relief from Allah. *"Indeed, Allah is with the patient."* (Quran 8:46). *"Seek God (Allah)'s help with patient perseverance and prayer. It is indeed hard, except for those who are humble"* (Quran 2:45). *"Be sure We shall test you with something of fear and hunger, some loss in goods, lives, and the fruits of your toil. But give glad tidings to those who patiently persevere"* (Quran 2:155).

Sabr often comes hand in hand with the concept of "shukr" or gratitude. Research in positive psychology shows that gratitude is a universally rewarding process for increasing happiness and emotional well-being (Emmons & Crumpler, 2000). A study of Muslim students conducted by Noor (2016) investigated the benefits of employing an Islāmic-based expressive appreciation method on happiness and well-being levels. The results showed that Islāmic-based gratitude increased the participant's happiness level due to the resonance it had with their beliefs and values compared with those practising a secular-based gratitude exercise and those who did not practice gratitude. The study concluded that Muslims engaging in sabr and shukr while making "dhikr" (remembrance of God, meditation) and taking actions based on their values are likely to experience increased levels of well-being and contentment.

The Guest House poem by the thirteenth-century Sufi Jalaluddin Rumi (Barks & Moyne, 2004) embodies the essence of acceptance and refers to the willingness to accept all unwanted experiences regardless of the associated discomfort. It can be a useful tool to defuse unhelpful thoughts as it creates a metaphor for life as a voyage filled with both pleasant and unwelcome experiences.

The central message is that whatever life's journey brings whether it is happiness or great difficulty, having faith and commitment to receive the experience without fear or aversion helps foster enlightenment and compassion towards the self and others. In life, we will inevitably experience both positive and negative situations. This duality of experiences is a natural facet of the human condition and serves to broaden our perspectives and deepen our understanding of the world around us. The bad experiences may be opportunities for growth while the good events are not necessarily conducive to spiritual and personal growth. *"But perhaps you hate a thing, and it is good for you, and perhaps you love a thing, and it is bad for you. And Allah Knows, while you know not"* (The Holy Quran 2:216).

Rumi uses metaphor and imagery to remind us that instead of resisting our thoughts and feelings, we should instead welcome them as if they were guests entering our home. In the poem, Rumi compares being human to being a guest house that welcomes our emotions. He likens our unexpected feelings to guests and notes that whether they are positive or negative, embrace them fully, as they serve to clear the way for new emotions and experiences to allow us to constantly evolve and grow.

The poem instils the hope that terrible things may happen, but there is always a good outcome when new feelings emerge. Welcome the feeling of sadness into your guest house with an open mind and heart. It is a way of trusting Allah even when you do not understand his plan.

The poem suggests that, when we resist challenging experiences, it only intensifies our discomfort and leads to the perception that the situation is permanent. Acceptance means that we do not just accept how life treats us, but we also accept the reaction that the situation may cause us to feel (Barks & Moyne, 2004). An example is then when we feel insulted by someone our natural response is to feel anger towards that person. Rather than pretending it is okay or repressing the anger, if we notice it and acknowledge it mindfully, then the power the anger has over us is reduced.

Similarly, thoughts and emotions also lose their power once we start to acknowledge them non-judgementally. The poem suggests that unwanted experiences arise and pass, but the key to our response is within ourselves. By accepting discomfort, we can ease the feeling of permanence and allow it to pass through us like a visitor who enters through the front door and exits through the back.

Cognitive Defusion

Cognitive defusion is a helpful technique that enables us to distance ourselves from our thoughts, images, and memories, allowing us to view them as passing experiences. Defusion skills can assist in recognizing negative thoughts and detaching from them rather than giving them power and belief. Cognitive fusion is when we believe our thoughts are true and become stuck in them, like a spider's web. This can prevent us from living a life based on values. Both Islām and ACT teach us to stand back from our thoughts, meta-cognitions, and actions so that we can live a fulfilling and meaningful life.

Cognitive fusion has parallels with the concept of "waswasa" which the Quran refers to as a state of persistent uncorroborated fears, worries, or "whispers." The Quran states *"and We have already created man and know what his self (nafs) whispers (waswasa) to him, and We are closer to him than [his] Jugular vein"* (Quran 50:16).

Just as ACT talks about creating perspective and separating fused content from the self, the Quran also recommends separating the self from the content of waswasa by using remembrance of God as this will increase proximity with the Almighty and bring ease: *"Verily in the remembrance of Allah, there is contentment of the heart"* (Quran 13:28). Therefore, using Islāmic techniques to help Muslims detach from their thoughts and get closer to Allah can be effective in motivating change. In ACT, defusion is often compared with the metaphor of the mind being akin to the sky, with thoughts resembling fleeting clouds that come and go. This aligns with a verse from the Quran and highlights that negative thoughts or feelings are temporary and not permanent. *"For indeed, with hardship will be ease"* (Quran 94.5).

Contact with the Present Moment

ACT encourages focus on what is happening in the present moment instead of being mired in worry and rumination. As internal and external events unfold, we engage in them without judgement, be they pleasant or unpleasant.

Being present in the moment can help with the management of pain by creating the mental space to detach from cognitive entanglement and develop tolerance and acceptance, rather than fighting unhelpful thoughts by engaging in them or trying to conquer them. The Holy Quran recommends awareness and remembrance as a way of creating peace. *"Those who have faith and whose hearts find peace in the remembrance of God- truly it is in the remembrance of God that hearts find peace"* (The Holy Quran 13:28).

When the mind is allowed space and silence, then any thoughts entering the mind should be considered exactly that, just thoughts, to be observed rather than be the defining factor of an individual's sense of self. In Islāmic practice, prayer and praise of God are used during challenging times to free ourselves from mental distress and find peace and balance. The Prophet Muhammed ﷺ advised a companion *"Be mindful of Allah and Allah will protect you. Be mindful of Allah and you will find Him in front of you"* (Hadith 19, 40 Hadith an-Nawawi).

Ibn al-Qayyim (691 AH to 751 AH) explained the concept of present-moment awareness as the *"continuous knowledge and conviction of the servant in the awareness of the Truth, glory be to Him, over his outward and inward states"* (Madārij al-Sālikīn 2/65) and *" to observe the heart, in awareness of the Truth, with every thought and step"* (Source: Madārij al-Sālikīn 2/66).

A pivotal principle in Islām is present-moment awareness without attachment to events of the past or worries about the future. The Islāmic practice of Muraqabah, which metaphorically means meditation, enables the individual to watch and take care of their soul and gain a closeness to their Creator. Muraqabah serves as a reminder that the Almighty is All-Seeing and All-Knowing. This leads to a heightened sense of awareness and presence in our actions, thoughts, feelings, and inner states of being. *"Surely Allah knows the unseen of the heavens and earth. And Allah is All-Seeing of what you do"* (Quran 49:18).

Those who are attempting to perfect their daily prayer discard their worldly problems and concerns and concentrate on each movement and recitation. When the mind wanders and they become troubled by their thoughts, feelings, or sensations, they are encouraged to return to what they are reciting without passing judgement on themselves for being mindless (Tanhan, 2019). Appreciating the Almighty's moment-by-moment creation by being present in mind is the path to experiencing the real meaning of life (the worship of Allah) and living it with true purpose.

The idea of "tawba," which means repentance or returning to the correct path, is vital for regaining present-moment awareness. It helps us break free from negative thoughts about our failures and motivates us to pursue actions that align with our values or have meaning. Tawba requires genuine intention and can be invoked anytime and anywhere at times of failure (Tahir, 2022). Prophet Muhammed ﷺ is reported to have said that the doors of tawba will remain open until the sun rises from the West. *"Verily, towards the Western sun is an open gate the length of which is seventy years of travel. It will remain open for repentance until the sun rises from there"* (Sunan Ibn Mājah 4070).

The Quran emphasizes the importance of not overwhelming the soul beyond its capacity, which serves as a source of encouragement and helps to promote resilience. The following verses in the Quran *"We burden not any person but that which he can bear"* (Quran 6:152) and *"Allah does not charge a soul except with that within its capacity"* (Holy Quran 2:286) encourage people who struggle to deal with life's challenges to pray as a method of cultivating a sense of presence (Hussain, 2011).

The Self as Context

Self as context refers to self-awareness or the "observing self," the part that notices thoughts, feelings, sensations, and the images that pass through our minds. Within the ACT model, "self as context" means recognising that our self is separate from our thoughts, emotions, or physical bodies and challenges our self-constructed identity or the "self as content," particularly when it prevents positive behavioural changes. Self as context can help people learn how to observe their pain without becoming their pain.

Within Islām, the nafs/self directs our being and tells us what to do, controls us, and dominates us (Yavuz et al., 2016). The nafs operates out of one of three states, Nafs al-Ammara, Nafs al-Lawwama, and Nafs al-Mutmainna which resonate, respectively, with self as content, self as process, and self as context. Nafs al-Ammara (commanding self) is the part of us that is caught up in unhelpful thoughts and becomes engrossed in self-stories which causes us to descend into negativity.

When the first nafs takes control, the Nafs al-Lawwama becomes active, and we develop an awareness that our feelings and actions are wrong which can then help us realise the importance of changing behaviours and acting in the service of long-term values. When change occurs, the Nafs al-Mmutmainna or the "calm centre" is triggered, and we experience a more stable sense of self and flexible perspective of our experience thereby achieving contentment and tranquillity. (Rothman & Coyle, 2018).

Learning to control the nafs (self) or the ego allows us to find direction to free ourselves from becoming attached to erroneous self-stories or limiting beliefs. The key to opening the door to self as context is present-moment awareness of thoughts and feelings without judgement. This helps cultivate a state of mind where the realities of both mental and emotional states become clear without getting lost in a sea of thoughts and sensations and helps develop the flexibility to use self-management techniques while maintaining a faith-based perspective.

Values

Chronic pain can cause people to seek quick and temporary relief, which may limit their ability to participate in important activities such as exercise, socializing, maintaining relationships, intimacy, and engaging in family and community events. Additionally, it may impact their ability to practice their faith and engage in prayer. A valued action is likely to be personal even though cultural, religious, and moral factors may underpin it. A values-based life can only be achieved when the individual commits to pursuing those values, even in adversity. The Muslim faith discourages avoidance behaviours in the face of an aversive experience or situation and encourages acting on values even when the natural urge is to avoid pain (Hussain, 2011).

The fatalistic view that "my pain is here to stay and nothing I do can change my suffering" can be challenged by using the Hadith, "*Trust in Allah but also tether your camel*" which reflects the idea that people should act and engage in self-management rather than resign to God for providing a solution (Edward-Moad, 2018).

There is a strong compatibility between the ACT concept of values and Islām (Yavuz et al., 2016). Islāmic guidance states that this world is temporary and fragile and that it is a preparation for the afterlife. How people conduct themselves during their life journey will determine their final destination. Thus, the goal may be to reach a successful afterlife, while the values-based actions in achieving this goal will be to live a life in the servitude of Allah. The Prophet Muhammed ﷺ described this as "*To worship Allah as if you see Him, and if you do not see Him, He sees you*" (Sahih Bukhari 4777).

Committed Actions

Committed action means living a productive and God-conscious life in line with our values while acknowledging that pain and difficulty are an unavoidable part of life. From this perspective, being observant and committed to pursuing values helps ensure a legacy based on actions as every Muslim is questioned upon these on the day of judgement. Thus, following moral, social, and behavioural principles is integral to committed actions.

The tombstone metaphor, often used in ACT to promote the motivation to living a values-based life, explores what people would want their life to stand for after they have left this world (Hayes et al., 2006). A valuable way to frame this for Muslims is to ask the individual what they would want to hear about themselves if they could attend their funeral. A Muslim's deeds are all they take with them when they leave this world and knowing that their life has been meaningful and full of virtuous deeds is a way to establish a lasting legacy that supports happiness in this world and the hereafter.

Within the ACT model, the absence of sadness is not a "normal" state, but, instead, pain, difficulties, and unpleasant experiences are inevitable and natural consequences of life (Hayes et al., 2012). Likewise, Islām acknowledges that pain or uncomfortable experiences are tests of life and are inevitably transient. For Muslims experiencing pain and suffering, this approach allows an appropriate rationale for the individual to take responsibility for their psychological and physical well-being, recognising that pain and suffering may be a test from the Almighty. However, it comes with the responsibility of taking committed action based on their values to alleviate suffering.

Indeed, Allah will not change the condition of a people until they change what is in themselves. And when Allah intends for a people ill, there is no repelling it.

(Quran 13:11)

Whenever a Muslim is afflicted by harm from sickness or other matters, God will expiate his sins, like leaves drop from a tree.

(Hadith from Bukhari and Muslim)

References

Barks, C., & Moyne, J. (2004). *Maulana Jalal Al-Din Rumi*. Harper San Francisco. ISBN 10: 0062509586; ISBN 13: 9780062509581

Biglan, A., Hayes, S. C., & Pistorello, J. (2008). Acceptance, and commitment: Implications for prevention science. *Prevention Science, 9*(3), 139–152. https://doi.org/10.1007/s11121-008-0099-4

Edward-Moad, O. (2018). *Tying your camel: An Islamic perspective on methodological naturalism*. Yaqeen Institute. https:// yaqeeninstitute.org/omar-

Emmons, R. A., & Crumpler, C. A. (2000). Gratitude as a human strength: Appraising the evidence. *Journal of Social and Clinical Psychology*, *19*, 56–69.

Hadith 19, 40 Hadith an Nawawi. https://sunnah.com/nawawi40:19

Harris, R. (2009). *ACT made simple: An easy-to-read primer*. New Harbinger Publications, Inc.

Harris, R. (2011). *Embracing your demons: An overview of acceptance and commitment therapy*. Psychotherapy.

Harris, R. (2019). *ACT made simple*. New Harbinger Publications, Inc.

Hayes, S. C. (2004). Acceptance and commitment therapy and the new behaviour therapies: Mindfulness, acceptance, and relationship. In S. C. Hayes, V. M. Follette & M. Linehan (Eds.), *Mindfulness and acceptance: Expanding the cognitive behavioural tradition* (pp. 1–29). Guilford.

Hayes, S. C. (2005). *Get out of your mind and into your life: The new acceptance and commitment therapy*. New Harbinger Publications.

Hayes, S. C., Luoma, J. B., Bond, F. W., Masuda, A., & Lillis, J. (2006). Acceptance and commitment therapy: Model, processes, and outcomes. *Behaviour Research and Therapy*, *44*(1), 1–25.

Hayes, S. C., Pistorello, J., & Levin, M. E. (2012). Acceptance and commitment therapy as a unified model of behaviour change. *The Counseling Psychologist*, *40*(7), 976–1002.

Hayes, S. C., Strosahl, K. D., & Wilson, K. G. (2004). *Acceptance and commitment therapy: An experiential approach to behavior change*. Paperback.

Hayes, S. C., Wilson, K. G., Gifford, E. V., Follette, V. M., & Strosahl, K. (1996). Experiential avoidance and behavioural disorders: A functional dimensional approach to diagnosis and treatment. *Journal of Consulting and Clinical Psychology*, *64*(6), 1152–1168.

Hernández-López, M., Cepeda-Benito, A., Díaz-Pavón, P., & Rodríguez-Valverde, M. (2021). Psychological inflexibility, and mental health symptoms during the COVID-19 lockdown in Spain: A longitudinal study. *Journal of Contextual Behavioral Science*, *19*, 42–49. https://contextualscience.org/applied_rft

Hussain, F. A. (2011). *Therapy from the Quran and Hadith*. A reference guide for character development. Darrusalam.

Ibn al Qayyim al Madaarij as-Saalikeen. www.hasbunallah.com.au/madarij-al-salikeen/

Noor, N. (2016). Effects of an Islamic-based gratitude strategy on Muslim students' level of happiness. *Mental Health Religion & Culture*, *19*(7), 686–703.

Pervez, A. (2014, December 30). *Sabr Key to Jannah*. http://messageinternational.org/sabr-is-key-to-jannah/

Rothman, A., & Coyle, A. (2018). Toward a framework for Islamic psychology and psychotherapy: An Islamic model of the soul. *Journal of Religion and Health*, *57*(5), 1731–1744. https://doi.org/10.1007/s10943-018-0651-x

Sahih al-Bukhari – A collection of hadith compiled by Imam Muhammad al-Bukhari Containing over 7500 hadith (with repetitions) in 97 books. https://sunnah.com/

Sahih al-Bukhari 4777, Book 65, Hadith 299 https://sunnah.com/bukhari:4777

Sunan Ibn Mājah 4070. www.abuaminaelias.com/dailyhadithonline/2021/05/21/sun-rises-west/

Tahir, R. (2022). *Repentance as a way of life: Islam, spirituality, & practice.* Published: August 6, 2018. Retrieved December 12, 2022, from https://yaqeeninstitute.org/ read/paper/repentance-as-a-way-of-life-islam-spirituality-practice

Tanhan, A. (2019). Acceptance and commitment therapy with ecological systems theory: Addressing Muslim mental health issues and wellbeing. *Journal of Positive Psychology and Wellbeing, 3*(2), 197–219. http://journalppw.com/index.php/JPPW/ article/view/172

Yavuz, F. K., Nieuwsma, J., Walser, R., Hayes, S., & Tan, S. (2016). ACT and Islam. In *ACT for clergy and pastoral counselors: Using acceptance and commitment therapy to bridge psychological and spiritual care,* New Harbinger (pp. 139–148).

https://sunnah.com/ibnmajah:4070

Part 2

5 Outline for a Six-Session Act Programme

Assessment Session – Managing Contingencies

Agenda

* Therapist orientation
* Rapport
* Risk management
* Chronic pain versus acute pain
* Client orientation

Therapist Orientation

Although, in previous chapters, people living with pain may have interchangeably been referred to as patients and clients, for the sake of simplicity, hereon, the person being treated will be referred to as the client and the one delivering the treatment as the therapist. The highlighted text in the subsequent chapters will contain scripted information for the client.

When starting to frame ACT From an Islāmic point of view, the aim is to help facilitate transformation that will increase faith in God and help develop hope and acceptance of the situation. When introducing Islāmic concepts to clients, it is important to avoid preaching as each client may have their own level of spirituality or religiosity. The goal is not to pass judgement on an individual's level of righteousness. Rather, to strive to assist individuals in reconnecting with their Islāmic values by utilizing the Islāmic framework. It is important to remind them that Islām is not just a religion, but a way of life.

During the sessions, individuals can explore how their cultural assumptions, rather than their Islāmic faith, may be contributing to unhelpful thoughts. By shifting their focus to Islāmic concepts, they may experience a decrease in distress and an improvement in their mindset and condition.

DOI:10.4324/9781003329626-7

The treatment described in this chapter is meant to ensure that the right processes are given the spotlight and delivered in a flexible way that adapts to the individual's presenting problems. Although the six processes have been described sequentially, ACT is not a linear technique. The sequence may work for some and not for others. The benefit of this is that the therapist can apply greater flexibility in their clinical work and fully engage with their client. For the client, they will learn and understand *healing isn't linear and struggles can occur at all stages*. Each process is delivered according to its relevance to the client.

Although it is important to be flexible in the order of addressing processes, having a structure for the sessions is necessary. The sessions are likely to last between 50 minutes to an hour. Furthermore, though the treatment is limited to six sessions, the therapist at their own discretion can choose to expand these depending on the client's engagement and presentation and pace the sessions accordingly.

Some of the processes may need to be repeated and reiterated. Each session will begin with checking in with the client's progress and picking up threads from the previous session to identify any emerging psychological themes. At the beginning of each session, the therapist must remind themselves to treat each client with compassion and genuine respect for their inherent ability to make change without focusing on trying to "fix" them or make judgements about the client.

It is important to remain humble and not promise the clients that their pain will be removed as this will lead to unrealistic expectations. The therapist's role is to work in the service of the client to help them improve the quality of their life with or without pain. As with any other intervention, while delivering ACT methods and exercises, it is vital not to lose sight of the importance of clinical skills around reflective listening, empathy, pace, and relationship building.

Managing Crisis

Whilst suicide is considered haram in the Islāmic religion, it is not uncommon to have clients with active suicidal ideation. During the assessment, it is essential to assess any risk factors without assumption or judgement and to provide emergency contact numbers before treatment begins. If an emergency arises, it is important to take the necessary measures to stabilise the patient and ensure the safety of those in danger, and a signpost for support and spiritual guidance if the client is willing.

Rapport

Developing rapport is the first important task for any intervention, as without a connection between therapist and client, any intervention is unlikely to be successful. The goal of developing a good rapport between the therapist and client is to develop mutual trust and respect and create an environment in which the client feels safe, thereby increasing the likelihood of a successful outcome.

The first step to the therapeutic journey is to allow the client to tell their "pain story" and listen with empathy while discussing their history of pain, specific areas of difficulties, functional issues, reasons for seeking therapy, and hopes and expectations. It is also an opportunity to normalise individual experiences and validate the importance of the experience of chronic pain and how their journey makes them the "expert" on their pain. The client's goals and expectations can be identified, and the aims of the intervention can be agreed based on the workability of the client's expectations. At this juncture, providing the client with some psychoeducation on the difference between acute and chronic pain and the neuroscience of pain is helpful.

Chronic Pain versus Acute Pain

Acute pain is typically due to an injury or illness. This pain serves as a warning system to alert us that something is wrong and to prevent further harm to our bodies. It is important to note that, regardless of where or how the pain is felt, it originates from the brain. The nerves in our body, including those in the spinal column and brain, adjust to our surroundings and actions. After the injury has healed, the pain usually subsides. Acute pain is often short in duration and is usually proportionate to the severity of the injury. It may take weeks or months to dissipate fully, depending on the nature of the injury. For example, a broken leg will take longer to heal than a sprain of the ankle.

It is important to know that chronic pain can last for more than three months and is not always a reliable indicator of an injury, even though an injury may have triggered it. Persistent pain that lingers beyond tissue healing (around 3–6 months) has more to do with a sensitive nervous system, which means the body stays in alarm mode even after tissues have healed. This leads to central sensitisation when the brain's alarm system overreacts to harmless or mild stimulation and increases pain intensity.

Chronic pain has two components: Primary pain, which refers to unpleasant sensations in the body, and secondary suffering, which is caused by the mental and emotional distress resulting from resistance and reactivity Our nerves can become sensitive depending on several factors such as exercise, diet, actions, emotions, beliefs, and environment. Neglecting proper exercise and maintaining an unhealthy diet can increase pain perception, as can erratic actions and negative emotions. Making conscious decisions and managing thoughts and emotions can reduce "pain volume." When the pain volume and perception are reduced, it is possible to begin the positive cycle of increasing activity, working towards personal goals, and changing our relationship with pain.

We know that making positive changes and engaging in enjoyable and valued activities releases happy chemicals, i.e., endorphins which boost our sense of agency and our motivation to effect positive change and help us pursue meaningful goals. Dwelling on limitations instead of appreciating what we can achieve restricts our ability to grow. If, for example, chronic pain has made it difficult to enjoy regular walks and exercise, rather than focusing on the loss of this activity, it may be helpful to look for alternative activities that are within our reach and may be just as enjoyable.

The assessment session finishes with orienting the client to the treatment being offered and how this approach teaches individuals to accept their thoughts, feelings, and struggles instead of resisting or feeling negative about their situation. It is also explained how this approach resonates with Islām.

Client Orientation

ACT is a therapeutic approach that aims to increase valued action in the presence of pain and suffering. This treatment is designed to help people with chronic pain and illness as well as those with emotional afflictions. Being physically ill or having a disability is difficult and stressful. We know that, when dealing with a physical condition, the problems extend far beyond physical health. People with pain may experience changes in their relationships, thoughts, and mood. Some question their identity and the significance and aim of their disease. Many people experience conflict in their religion and relationship with God.

This intervention aims to help you develop techniques for pain management using an evidence-based treatment that has been Islāmically adapted. It is an intervention that will help you navigate your difficulties using a framework that fits in with your religious background whilst also helping with practical ways of managing pain and increasing your quality of life.

These practical aspects of pain management will include developing psychological flexibility to help you learn to accept and live with pain by engaging in paced, value-based, goal-orientated activities that will help you separate from the presence of thoughts, feelings, and behaviours associated with pain and help you move forward towards your Islāmic values to create a meaningful life. Trials and suffering are part of life, as are joy and happiness. However, we have been sent guidance on how to deal with them through the Quran and the teachings of the Prophet Muhammed ﷺ which we will use throughout the sessions to help align you towards your values while using ACT as an evidence-based treatment.

The client will be informed about the number of planned sessions, and the time and date for each session will be mutually agreed upon.

6 Treatment Session 1

Agenda

- Review of the assessment session
- Introduce creative hopelessness
- Sabr and acceptance
- Breathing exercise

In the first treatment session, check in with the client about how they found the assessment session and whether they had any thoughts or reflections they may want to share. This session aims to move the client towards a state of "creative hopelessness" and to help determine what options exist if pain elimination is not attainable.

Many clients mention avoidance as a coping mechanism, such as skipping exercise, limiting domestic chores, stopping work, declining social invitations, avoiding prayer, no longer attending the mosque, and so on. Creative hopelessness helps clients reassess their goals and values by helping them identify how they may have been avoiding their pain and evaluate what that avoidance has cost them. The client can also be directed to reflect on the success or failure of prior pain management approaches they may have used to help motivate them to try new strategies.

> **Example:**
>
> You may have tried different ways to get rid of the pain and suffering; some things may have helped, while others not so much. Using strategies that have not helped can feel like your head is banging against a brick wall and must be frustrating. Let us try to understand what works for you and what does not. Some questions that may help with this process are as follows:

DOI:10.4324/9781003329626-8

What do you want in life?*It is common for clients to say, "I just want to be free of the pain" or "If I didn't have this pain, I could be doing much more with my life."*

How would you live your life differently if you knew that your pain would never go away?*Many people live in the hope of removing pain in their lives, but once they start accepting that pain is there to stay, this can help them move towards engaging in activities they may have been avoiding.*

What have you been doing so far to ease the pain?*With this question, we can identify what behaviours and strategies the client has been using to manage the pain and pivot towards how helpful or unhelpful those methods may have been.*

Worksheet 1.1 has some examples of cost benefits and can help the client identify what strategies they have been using and whether they have been helpful or not.

Carrying out an analysis of prior treatments or strategies employed by the client to control pain is a helpful way to identify short- and long-term benefits of coping behaviours and the consequences of their actions. It is the starting point to help motivate the client to consider that they may need to change direction and explore what is important for them and what they want their life to look like. The client can be supported to shift their thinking towards an

Worksheet 1.1 Identifying Cost Benefits of Pain Coping Strategies

Type of pain management	Short-term gains	Long term	Effect on quality of life
Taking a cocktail of painkillers daily	It eases the pain for a while	No change in pain – pain is still steady and constant	Often makes me feel drowsy and less inclined to do anything
Avoidance of exercise	Stops pain from flaring up	Muscles have become stiff and unconditioned	More avoidance of activities
Avoiding family events	Reduces anxiety	People have stopped inviting me to events	Feel alone and neglected
Avoiding daily prayers	Less chance of triggering pain and discomfort	A slight change in pain over the long term. Pain still flares up	Constant feelings of guilt and worry about letting myself and God down

alternative perspective by first validating their attempts to manage their pain and then asking some key probing questions:

How has that worked for you? When addressing the client's examples of what they have been doing to manage their pain, the goal here is to be inquisitive rather than critical. The client can be provided with a blank worksheet to complete their own cost/benefit analysis (Appendix 1). Some questions that can guide the client to explore their behaviours are as follows:

- What is the cost of these behaviours?
- How much time do you spend doing these behaviours?
- What have you lost?
- What have you given up?
- Is it making your life bigger or smaller?

Summarise the difficulties the client may have faced while using various strategies to manage chronic pain, including what the client wants and what they have been doing or not doing due to the fear of aggravating pain. It is useful to ask about other things they have tried to minimize the impact of pain on their lives such as taking herbal remedies or seeking spiritual remedies.

This discussion may evoke emotional reactions such as sadness, fear, and frustration when people realise that they have been trying so hard to cope with pain but with little benefit. Validating the client's feelings and emphasising their feelings as a normal reaction are helpful. Rather than being critical of previous treatments, use the information to generate a discussion on what alternative options may exist. Ask the question:

"What does your experience tell you?" This question can elicit the client's willingness to move towards a different path and develop acceptance of their chronic pain condition if pain elimination is not achievable. The focus on long-term consequences rather than immediate positive outcomes such as experiential avoidance of aversive situations helps to shift the client's agenda from pain control to pain management.

Ask the client to consider two options: One in which they have less pain and stress but none of the other valued life dimensions, and two, they continue to experience pain and stress symptoms but also have a quality of life which encompasses their desirable valued dimensions.

The most powerful catalyst for the client's willingness to try something different is their realisation that the struggle to control or keep away from situations has been feeding their pain, rather than making it better. They are then more likely to be motivated to make changes that align with their personal and religious values because they become more hopeful about breaking out of the feeling of "stuckness." The client's struggle with pain can be moved towards acceptance by using metaphors to illustrate how trials and tribulations are part of Allah's power, grace, and justice.

Metaphors in ACT are a powerful way of helping the client understand how feelings and thoughts can influence actions. The Islāmic perspective of sabr (patience) functions to enable a willingness to accept unwanted inner or external experiences. However, sabr does not imply that we accept suffering, deny our emotions, or remain passive to our difficulties. Sabr is a way of developing acceptance, but it is important not to use sabr as an excuse to become passive.

For example, one form of acceptance is passively resigning to life's afflictions which removes agency and leads to experiential avoidance to avoid aggravating the pain condition. An example might be that of a person who spends all day in bed because their life is dominated by attempts to escape from or eliminate pain or they may adopt the sick role and rely on family to do everything for them. A good example of sabr without passivity is illustrated in the story of Hajar, the wife of Prophet Ibrahim (AS).

When Allah instructed Ibrahim (AS) to leave his wife and their baby in the barren desert, he trusted Allah's plan and so did Hajar. She understood that Ibrahim (AS) was following Allah's orders and believed that whatever Allah had planned was for the best. However, when Ibrahim (AS) left her behind and her thirsty baby started to cry relentlessly, she did not sit passively even though she had sabr and trust in Allah. Instead, she did something to try and help herself. Hajar ran from the mountains of Safa and Marwa not once but seven times to try to find water for her crying baby. When she could not find any water Hajar prayed for Allah's help. Allah answered her prayer and the zam zam spring burst forth from the ground. Hajar's actions are called *sa'i* which in Arabic means striving and subsequently became one of the rituals for performing the Hajj pilgrimage. The lessons that Hajar teaches in her actions is that in times of tribulations, and suffering it is important to have optimism (through thinking good of Allah), Tawakkul (having reliance on Allah), Sabr (having patience), and Taqwa (being God-conscious).

Another metaphor that can illustrate acceptance, perseverance, and endurance is that of the cactus plant. In desolate environmental conditions, the cactus perseveres to survive by pushing its roots deep into the soil to find the invisible underground streams to store water for difficult days. When in the depths of despair, we can purify the soul by practising patience, gratitude, and a willingness to act on our values. "*Oh, you who believe! Seek help with patient perseverance and prayer, for God is with those who patiently persevere*" (Quran 2:153).

The Guest House poem by Rumi is often used by ACT practitioners and can also be used to help the client move towards acceptance using an Islāmic stance to pain and suffering. Introduce the Guest House poem to the client as a metaphor describing life's journey and how we can appreciate the uncertainty of life and embrace difficulties.

Rumi tells us that, instead of resisting our thoughts and feelings, we should welcome them as if they were guests entering our home because we humans are like a guest house in which we accommodate our emotions whether they are wanted or unwanted. The poem explains how undesired experiences arise and pass, but the key to overcoming discomfort is within us.

If we accept each unpleasant thought and emotion as a temporary visitor and embrace it with openness and acknowledge that each experience is sent to us by Allah for a reason, then the fear of that discomfort being permanent eases and we can allow it to pass over us like a visitor who comes in through the front door and leaves through the back.

Instead of resisting our thoughts and feelings, we should welcome them as though they were guests who are sent to us from the Divine to clear out the emotional overload held by our body and to make way for new emotions and experiences. This poem tells us that in times of trials and tribulations even when we do not understand Allah's plan we should practice sabr and put trust in Allah's decree knowing that in the end it will be worth it.

We can also see this through the word *alhamdulillah*, one of the most common and powerful words that Muslims use in all conditions regardless of pleasant or unpleasant experiences/situations. For Muslims, gratitude to Allah is a way of life and helps us retain a perpetual sense of optimism. By praising and thanking Allah for all His blessings regardless of the situation being good or bad we are affirming that behind every difficulty there is divine wisdom and a great reward for being patient. The Quran tells us *"And be patient, for indeed, God does not allow the rewards of those who do good to go to waste"* (Quran: 11:115).

This discussion touches upon the process of acceptance without using the word acceptance. Sometimes, acceptance may come in the form of passively resigning to life's afflictions which removes agency and leads to experiential avoidance to avoid aggravating the pain condition. Remind the client that Islām encourages value-based actions even when faced with aversive situations. This means that it is important for the client to avoid using acceptance as an excuse to become passive.

Furthermore, if a client believes that life can only be enjoyed if the pain is removed from their life, they may avoid activities such as socialisation, exercise, and prayer and rely on medication to fight the pain. Being heavily medicated may reduce pain, but it will limit the ability to engage in valued activities. This can create a tug of war to control the uncontrollable, effectively leading to life becoming smaller and more limited for that person as valued activities become scarce.

A healthier form of acceptance is for those who neither succumb to their affliction nor focus on eradication but instead are active and responsive and develop different behaviour patterns and habits to adjust to the different demands of persistent pain. They learn to understand how to soothe themselves from pain and discomfort without compromising their values.

Examples might be adapting the prescribed salah prayer movements to be carried out while sitting on a chair instead of avoiding prayer, pacing when engaging in exercise or domestic chores, or visiting family for shorter periods rather than avoiding them completely.

The natural response to aversive situations is to turn away from that experience or engage in experiential avoidance. This may not always be a bad thing, but it is harmful when we pull away from valued activities. Experiential avoidance can end up being akin to driving around a circular junction and avoiding exiting the junction because of the fear of pain being triggered. This behaviour is not only a short-term solution but can intensify the experience that you might be trying to avoid ending up in being looped into a cycle of psychological suffering.

When we learn acceptance, we open ourselves up and make room for our thoughts, feelings, and sensations without fighting or running from them, or allowing them to control what we do or do not do.

In the next session, we will practice an exercise referred to as "dropping an anchor" which is a useful tool to help cultivate acceptance as it allows the space to manage pain and emotions. It is common for people with chronic pain to become helpless with an inability to control pain-related thoughts and sensations while anticipating the flare-up of pain. This often leads to the magnification of the threat value of the pain and leads to further distress. This exercise can help us stay with the difficult experience and learn to accept the experience without the struggle to get rid of it.

Summarise the learnings of the session, and before ending, introduce a deep breathing exercise that the client can also practice independently over the week. However, before carrying out the breathing practice, educate the client on the neuroscience of deep breathing and its relevance to supporting pain management as knowing the purpose and benefits of deep breathing techniques will help to increase their motivation to practice the exercise.

Before we end today's session, we are going to learn a deep breathing exercise but before that, I would like to explain the mechanics of this so you are clear about how this exercise can help you.

Research shows that controlled breathing improves relaxation and, as a result, reduces the perception of pain. Slowing and deepening our breathing is known to reduce the perception of pain. When we feel acute or chronic pain, it sets off a series of reactions in the body. The pain triggers our "fight or flight" response in the central nervous system (CNS) as the brain identifies the pain as a danger signal. Stress hormones like cortisol are released into the bloodstream, and breathing tends to become shallow. Our bodies become tense, tightening our muscles, making the pain worse. When we try to fight pain, we experience an increase in tension and stress, which causes the pain signals to rise. Working with the breath helps us to reduce the stress reaction and helps to shift us out of the fight-or-flight response. By taking a moment to engage in conscious breathing, the body relaxes, and the tension around the pain site is released. Deep breathing can help ease the pain to a level where we feel we have more control and agency over our responses. So, whether you are overwhelmed due to physical pain, or emotionally, breathing deeply can help you achieve a sense of calm. It just takes five minutes daily to practice deep breathing. We will end our session today with a deep breathing exercise which we will practice at the end of each session to help build your confidence.

Instructions for Deep Breathing

Deep Breathing Exercise

Sit comfortably, or if you prefer, lie down. Start by noticing your breathing; pay attention to how you are breathing, and gently slow down your breathing. We are going to take deep breaths through the nose and exhale out through the mouth. The exhale will be longer and slower than the inhale. Place one hand on your abdomen and the other hand on your upper chest. Focus your breathing on your abdomen. As you breathe inhale to a count of five, and the hand on your abdomen should rise. Your abdomen should look like a balloon being inflated. Hold for three seconds and breathe out (exhale) to the count of eight, slowly through your mouth with pursed lips as though you are blowing out a candle. The abdomen should become flat against the spine like a balloon that is deflated. Your hand on your upper chest should make little movement while the other hand should correspond with the abdomen being inflated and deflated. Take slow and gentle breaths. As you gently build this rhythm and your breathing finds a comfortable speed, focus your mind on Allah. Carry on breathing like this for about five minutes, and as you finish, take one last deep inhale, and breathe out with a long and sharp breath. Just take a moment to notice how you feel.

The key is first to master the breathing technique to calm the CNS and then to connect to the divine with dhikr. Practice this breathing technique two to three times a day for 5–10 minutes. This natural breathing technique helps reduce pain intensity and manage pain spasms and is helpful for emotional regulation at times of stress and anxiety. You will get the most benefit if you practice this regularly as part of your daily routine.

Give the client a printed handout of the breathing exercise to encourage them to practice until the next session (Handout 2.1, Appendix 2).

7   Treatment Session 2

Agenda

- Homework review
- Present-moment awareness
- Values exercise, behaviour change, and goals
- Deep breathing exercise

Begin by reflecting on the previous session and how the client found the deep breathing exercise. The agenda for this session will be to follow up on the last session to cultivate acceptance using a grounding exercise to help the client stay present in the moment. The session will also use a values exercise to help the client identify goals and values to enable positive behaviour change.

The client may have found the breathing exercise difficult because it may feel unfamiliar and burdensome. If the client does not notice any benefit straight away, they may also lose motivation and faith in its value. Reiterate the purpose of the deep breathing exercise and remind the client that the key is perseverance. Using the analogy of learning to ride a bike or drive is helpful as once the client has practised the breathing technique to the point that it becomes easy and automatic, they will never forget what they have learned and will always be able to use it whenever they need it.

In the last session, we discussed how chronic pain can lead to avoidance behaviours and other unhelpful strategies to manage pain such as control and distraction. We discussed how sabar can help us move towards a state of acceptance and a willingness to pivot towards our values and goals.

A useful tool that we can use to help bring us back to a state of present-moment awareness especially if we are overwhelmed by pain and distress is the "dropping anchor" exercise. This exercise helps

DOI:10.4324/9781003329626-9

to facilitate a change from being controlling and distracting to being mindful and accepting of the present moment as it is.

Dropping Anchor – This exercise can be remembered by using the acronym ACE.

A: Acknowledge your thoughts and feelings
C: Come back into your body
E: Engage in what you are doing

Let us think about the pain right now and the struggle it might be creating for you.

First, acknowledge your thoughts and feelings, sensations, or urges that you may be experiencing with curiosity but without any judgement. For example, "I am noticing a thought that my pain is going to become worse" or "I am noticing some anxiety."

Second, come back into your body and connect with your physical body. You can do this by using the following strategies:

Slowly push your feet onto the floor and feel the ground beneath you; straighten your back or sit forward in your chair; slowly stretch your arms or neck and shrug your shoulders; press the tips of your fingers together.

Take a deep slow breath!

The important thing is that you do not try to avoid feelings or pain. Instead, you should stay aware of them and acknowledge that they are there. At the same time, be aware of your body as you move it.

Third, engage in what you are doing. Keep your attention on your thoughts and feelings and connect with your body by using your senses to notice five things you can see, four things you can hear, three things you can feel, two things you can smell, and one thing you can taste. This helps to ground you in the present.

By practising ACE regularly, it is possible to sit with the pain and accept it as it happens because you are no longer trying to fight it (Handout 2.2, Appendix 2).

Ask the client how the exercise made them feel. Elaborate on how noticing, naming, normalising, and giving purpose to their pain condition can open space for them to an awakening that will enable them to be receptive to seeking values-based goals rather than being overcome by fear and emotions that create misalignment with their fitrah.

The Quran stresses that trials and tribulations reconnect the individual with their fitrah and to the Almighty, thereby allowing us to reflect on our previous disposition and the blessings we have. Through the process of faith, patience, gratitude, and presence of mind, we can learn to unpack the experience of chronic pain and embark on a journey of spiritual reawakening and inner development.

Remind the client that the purpose of treatment is to allow them to engage in meaningful activities to improve their quality of life. Identifying values is the first step towards helping the client to think about the goals they want to set themselves to achieve a life where they can live with chronic pain but still have a quality of life that is adequate for their needs and congruent with their values.

What is really important to you? As life in this world is temporary, what direction would you choose for your life journey?

This question will help the client identify what values are important to them and whether they want to commit to a life based on their values and religious beliefs. Clients who become stuck in symptoms of pain and stress may find it emotionally taxing to identify their values and aspirations, especially if they believe that they are not realistic.

The Quran is a guide to help us lead a value-based, meaningful quality of life. *"There is no disease that Allah has created, except that He also has created its treatment"* (Sahih Al Bukhari 5678). Being in pain can often make us move away from our true purpose and meaning and create a disconnect from our values. Values are personal ethics or ideals that guide us to make decisions about the direction we may wish our life to take and reflect how we want to live not how we want to feel or think.

We cannot choose everything that happens to us, but we can choose how we react to different situations. Connecting with our values can help us live a life based on what we believe is right. Islām guides us to live a valued based life to benefit us in this world and the hereafter. Our values define what we want to stand for, how we want to relate to the rest of the world, and how we want to be remembered when we leave this temporary world. Values are the compass that helps us on the journey to achieve our goals and can relate to any aspects of our life such as health, finances, family, relationships, hobbies, and our relationship with Allah.

For Muslims, the concept of well-being transcends beyond this world into the hereafter. Therefore, the client's values are likely to reflect this.

For example, if the client's value is to live a life of compassion and care for others, their goal may be to dedicate their time to a charitable organization in servitude of the needy and less fortunate. However, if chronic pain and illness thwart the goal of working for a charitable organization, it does not mean they have to abandon their value of being compassionate towards others. Instead, the client may support the charity by attending fundraising events and showing kindness and compassion with their neighbours, friends, and so forth. Values are not about achieving any specific goal or success as we cannot always control whether we will reach our goals; however, our actions can be guided by our values even if our goals are not met.

Worksheet 1.2 can be used as an example to elicit the values the client has been moving away from and what may be preventing them from living in accordance with their values.

Step 1: Think of an activity or relationship in your life that you value, but that you have found yourself moving away from due to pain. It is a relationship you care a lot about or a spiritual activity, but you have noticed you are not as interested in it as you used to be.

Step 2: In the left box, write down what you value in that relationship or activity. How would you like to increase your valued activities?

Step 3: In the right box, write what difficult thoughts and feelings come up when you start taking action towards that value.|

Worksheet 1.2 Identifying Values Worksheet (Appendix 1)

Value	**Difficult thoughts/feelings/behaviour**
1. *To spend more time doing activities with my children and being a good mother.*	1. *I feel irritable and intolerant of them because I am in pain.*
2. *To be able to pray regularly and fulfil my religious duties.*	2. *The pain is too much and stops me from praying. Then I feel guilty.*
3. *Being a caring wife and companion to my husband.*	3. *I feel anxious all the time because I am no longer a good wife because of the pain.*
4. *To visit my parents more often and spend time with them as they are old and need my support.*	4. *I find it difficult to tolerate other people when I am in pain and become angry and irritable. I'm worried I might say something to upset them.*

Spend five minutes or so explaining this exercise. Validate the client's initial responses and encourage them to ponder on their own values and how they may have neglected them in the pursuit of gaining short-term relief from pain. Encourage the client to notice where they may feel "stuck" and how bad that experience feels.

For example, the client may be using avoidance strategies to stop flare-ups or tell themselves that the pain is there because they are a bad person. They may be using strong dosages of medication for pain elimination at the cost of living their life in the enjoyment of the blessings they still have. Avoidance behaviours that prevent the client from fully engaging in their life may sever their relationship with family, friends, and, more importantly, God.

Values in Islām promote and regulate behaviour to the benefit of society and its individuals, as well as to ensure a successful afterlife. A useful exercise to help the client clarify what they want their life to stand for is to ask them to imagine what statements they would want their loved ones, close friends, family, and acquaintances to make about them when they hear they have died. This exercise can be powerful in differentiating *desires* (for example, to be happy, pain-free, rich, and successful) from *values* (e.g., to be a kind loving parent, trustworthy friend, pious, and compassionate towards others). This is significant in light of the Islāmic belief that our deeds will accompany us in death.

Living a life based on values is a form of worship, and if the goal is to please the Almighty, then we would achieve this by living a life where we fulfil acts of worship. The Quran's description of the purpose of a Muslim's life is "*I have not created men except that they should serve Me*" (Quran: 56:51).

The term worship is inclusive in that it is not just following the five pillars of Islām but everything that an individual says or does to please Allah, including behaviours and actions. Our values are important because our actions as Muslims are intrinsically based on a desire to please our Lord.

When we align our values with the desire to please Allah, He will provide us with the drive to work continuously towards our goals without having expectations for the results. We may have control over our efforts, but Allah has complete power over the outcome and only expects us to act with pure intention because that is what we will be rewarded for, not the outcome. When we put our trust in Allah, it is easier to accept whatever life throws at us.

> **How is the way you are managing pain hindering you from your relationship with Allah?**

Ask the client to give examples of when they may have been so preoccupied with trying to control the uncontrollable that they may have drifted from their connection with Allah. The struggle with chronic pain often leads to values-based activities being avoided or neglected. An example of this might be a person who may be so preoccupied with trying to eliminate pain that they neglect their prayers, and community gatherings related to their spirituality and faith.

Remind the client that Islām views pain and suffering as a test not only to turn to Allah with trust but also to take decisive action when needed. Faith gives adversity and suffering significance because we are trusting in Allah's mercy, wisdom, and strength. Faith is like muscle tissue; the more it is stretched, the stronger it becomes. When tested through illness and pain, if we remain steadfast in the belief that Allah knows best and has not forsaken us, then the result is greater strength and capacity to endure. Prayer can help transform the feelings generated from dread and anguish into a sense of safety, hope, and optimism.

Remind the client that Allah promises us that He will be with us and guide us so long as we seek his assistance *"And your Lord say call on Me; I will answer your (prayer)"* (Quran: 40:60). Pain can often overwhelm us so much that we start drowning in a sea of hopelessness that we forget that we can still swim towards our spiritual shore and save ourselves.

It is important to point out to the client that prayer complements therapeutic intervention but does not replace effort and hard work to self-manage. *"Seek help with patient perseverance and prayer, for God is with those who patiently persevere"* (Quran: 2:153). Asking someone to rely on prayer alone without taking any positive steps to help themselves is ineffective.

It is not unusual for Muslim clients to adopt a fatalistic perspective, believing that their suffering is inevitable and beyond their control, or that it is their obligation as Muslims to accept Allah's will without complaining or asking for assistance. This mindset removes them from the responsibility of taking care of their health. The Quran states *"Man will not get anything unless he works hard"* (Quran 53:39).

This verse can help generate a discussion on the importance of striving to do what we can to help ourselves so that if we fail to achieve our goals, we know it is *qadar* (divine will) and not due to lack of effort. The Prophet Muhammed ﷺ said we should not suffer with silence and apathy but seek help through prophetic medicine.

Therefore, while it is important to accept afflictions with sabr (patience), it is also necessary to avoid passivity and inaction if we want to improve our overall quality of life and functioning. The Prophet ﷺ taught us by the example of his own life that this world is full of health and wealth-related challenges and unimaginable hardships. "*If Allah wants to do good to somebody, He afflicts him with trials*" (Sahih Bukhari 5645). He ﷺ advocated a holistic approach to the treatment of ill health by addressing the client's physical, mental, and spiritual state incorporating faith, gratitude, diet and nutrition, exercise, and dhikr.

Using verses from the Quran can help motivate the client to consider making changes that will help them move out of a state of inaction into a willingness to pivot towards change. "*Verily never will Allah change the condition of a people until they change it themselves (with their own souls)*" (Quran 13:11). "*And certainly, We shall test you with something of fear, hunger, loss of wealth, lives, and fruit, but give glad tidings to the patient, who when disaster strikes them, say, Indeed we belong to Allah, and indeed to him we will return*" (Quran: 2: 55–156). Prophet Muhammad ﷺ said, "*No fatigue, nor disease, nor sorrow, nor sadness, nor hurt, nor distress befalls a Muslim, even if it were the prick he receives from a thorn, but that Allah expiates some of his sins for that*" (Sahih Bukhari 5641).

Continue to reiterate that health and illness are a test for Muslims as well as a way of atoning for their sins. "*Whenever a Muslim is afflicted by harm from sickness or other matters, God will expiate his sins, like leaves drop from a tree*" (Sahih al-Bukhari 5647). This concept can be further elaborated when the ACT process of present-moment awareness is explored in subsequent sessions.

One of the companions of the Prophet ﷺ asked him why we should seek treatment when we have faith that Allah will heal us. Muhammad ﷺ replied "O *servants of God, seek treatment. Verily, Allah did not send a disease but that He also sent its treatment or cure*" (Sahih Bukhari 5678). The Prophet Muhammad ﷺ made it clear that every sickness has a corresponding treatment, and while this may not mean a cure for chronic pain, there is a possibility of living a meaningful life despite the ongoing presence of pain.

To enable the client to reflect on the need to balance action while letting go of things out of their control a well-known Hadith about having tawakkul and faith in Allah while taking concerted action can be used as a metaphor to expand the discussion about the importance of taking action to help ourselves regardless of the situation.

A Bedouin man left his camel without tying it. He was asked by the Prophet Muhammad ﷺ why he had not tethered the camel. The Bedouin responded that he was putting his trust in Allah. The Prophet ﷺ then replied, "*Tether your camel first, and then put your trust in Allah*" (Sunan al-Tirmidhi 2517).

This Hadith reflects the idea that we should act and engage in self-management rather than take the fatalistic view of relying on God alone to provide a solution. This means putting focus on what we can realistically control without being passive, and trusting that whatever the outcome, whether positive or negative, it is Allah's plan for the best. There is wisdom in letting go of things we cannot control so long as we have acted on what is in our control. Hence, we tie our proverbial camels and act where we can and with the rest, trust in Allah's plan. Trusting in Allah's plan is having tawakkul and is integral to Islām.

In Islām, we are responsible for taking care of our bodies and minds which includes seeking treatment appropriately not just for our physical health but also our mental health. This is knowing that, no matter what obstacles we may face, we have choices in life to take appropriate actions to help ourselves through advice and treatment. By seeking help and support to improve what you can do and how you feel and by finding a balance between the needs of the body and the soul, it is possible to learn to live with chronic pain with tawakkul.

When we are putting hope and trust in Allah, we must also endeavour to do our best to improve our lives by taking advice from professionals, increasing self-care, and adapting our lifestyle as best as we can because then we can find solace in knowing that we did what we could, and the rest is up to the *qadr* (decree) of Allah.

Once the client is able to define their chosen values, the next step is for the client to set themselves goals. Setting goals is about identifying what we would like to be able to do and how we can set out to achieve them. Setting personal and meaningful goals is a powerful way to improve quality of life and increase a sense of control. Goals move us from stagnation into the space of productivity. Many clients avoid moving towards their valued direction because they are avoiding pain and believe they have physically painful barriers that will stop them from reaching their goals.

The Prophet Muhammad ﷺ said, "*There are two blessings which many people do not make the most of and thus lose out: good health and free time*" (Sahih al-Bukhari 6412). Goal setting negates the illusion that we have ample energy, time, and resources and can prevent procrastination because it helps us manage our time better and gives us a purpose to act accordingly. It also brings meaning to life and improves motivation. The client is embarking on the road towards acceptance, knowing that the pain is here to stay, but life does not have to come to a standstill.

Inform the client that goals can be achieved in a gradual manner. Help the client set themselves some small achievable goals or some SMART goals as a homework exercise. Provide the client with the goal-setting handout to help them develop SMART goals to be discussed in the next session (Worksheet 1.3). As the session ends, finish off with the abdominal breathing exercise.

After the client has been reoriented to the session, reiterate the need for them to continue practising the deep breathing exercise as homework and to complete the goal-setting worksheet (Worksheet 1.3, Appendix 1).

References

Jami` at-Tirmidhi 2517 Book 37, Hadith 103, Vol. 4, Book 11, Hadith 2517, https:// sunnah.com/tirmidhi:2517

Sahih al-Bukhari 5645. https://sunnah.com/bukhari:5645

Sahih Bukhari 5641 https://sunnah.com/bukhari:5641

Sahih al-Bukhari 5647 Book 75, Hadith 7 https://sunnah.com/bukhari:5647

Sahih al-Bukhari 5678 Book 76, Hadith 1 https://sunnah.com/bukhari:5678

Sahih al-Bukhari 6412 Book 81, Hadith 1 https://sunnah.com/bukhari/81/1

8 Treatment Session 3

Agenda

- Homework review
- Goal setting and committed action
- Boom and bust
- Tawba and gratitude
- Introduction to thought defusion
- Deep breathing exercise

Begin the session with a review of the homework and any reflections on the last session. Discuss any further thoughts on values and goal setting. Within this session, the client's goals should be further clarified by referring to the goal setting Worksheet 1.3 which they were given in the last session (Appendix 2). Ask the client to choose two or three areas where there are significant discrepancies between their intentions and their activities and which areas they wish to work on to align their actions with their intentions. This might be physical activity, family life, or spiritual development and fulfilling their religious obligations. Providing an Islāmic perspective on goal setting can increase the client's motivation.

> Goal setting in pursuit of a purpose in life can be understood as the Sunnah of Allah Almighty. Allah had a goal-oriented agenda when he bestowed the message of Islām to the Prophet Muhammed ﷺ. The long-term vision was to spread Allah's word of Islām, but it took the implementation of short-term goals over decades to achieve the final goal and create a Muslim Ummah.
>
> We can just look at the exemplary life of Prophet Muhammed ﷺ who not only set the goal to complete the immense Islāmic mission bestowed upon him but was also engaged in a wide repertoire of other activities. These included social, domestic, business, family, and community responsibilities while at the same time carrying the heavy duty

DOI:10.4324/9781003329626-10

of being the custodian of the Quran and protector of the scribes. His goals were implemented during times of great tests and tribulations. Even though our life plans may feel insignificant in comparison, by following the sunnah and setting and achieving goals in a measured manner, we will be living our life according to Allah's sunnah.

You can reflect on your life and think about what goals you want to set. These could be in any domain whether it is physical, spiritual, intellectual, or social. For example, if your goal is to develop your spirituality, you need to identify your baseline and set some short-term goals to gradually reach the spiritual state you wish to be in. This may include adapting exercise regimes, family activities, prayer routines, daily Quran recitation, and dhikr to gradually build on the practice.

Sometimes, it is easier to avoid activities than to face the fear of aggravating pain. However, Allah tells us in Surah Al- Kahf *"And say not of anything, 'I am going to do it tomorrow.' Unless Allah should will"* (Quran 18:24–25). This verse highlights the importance of focusing on today and acting now rather than leaving things for tomorrow as tomorrow may never come. We can start with having trust in Allah to assist us on the journey to achieve our goals. Once we set goals that are closely aligned with our values, then regardless of the outcome, we have an opportunity to develop as a person. Even if the long-term goal is not achieved, there is always a valuable lesson behind that experience that will help us grow.

This explanation can lead to a discussion about the tendency to set goals/actions that are unrealistic or poorly defined. Encourage the client to set goals that are realistic and attainable, with a timeline and a clear intention to put in the effort and have trust in Allah. In other words, goals need to be SMART which stands for Specific, Measurable, Achievable, Realistic, and Timely. The client can be asked to define their goal using this strategy.

For example, if a client sets the goal to increase their engagement with family members, the therapist's role will be to support them to think about pacing themselves and increasing the activity in a graded and timed manner so as not to aggravate the pain or become exhausted.

Introduce the idea of exposure so that the client understands that to move towards a valued direction, they must be willing to feel the discomfort of the symptoms they have been working so hard to avoid. Check their commitment towards taking values-based actions even though it means exposure to discomfort.

For example, if a client sets the goal to increase their engagement with family members, support them to think about pacing themselves and increasing the activity in a graded and timed manner so as not to aggravate the pain or become exhausted. The Holy Quran states that, for change to be implemented effectively without overwhelming the individual, it is important to act in a paced and graded manner. An example of this is when Allah implemented the total prohibition of alcohol by revealing guidance in three separate chapters of the Quran in graded steps to enable successful change to be achieved (Quran 2:219, 4:43, 5:90).

Once we set goals for ourselves, the next step is to take committed action. It is easy to drift away from faith, life, and what is important to you when living with chronic pain. At times, you may feel stuck and unsure of what to do next but ultimately it is up to you to decide the next step. You can either stay as you are or make plans to change your life with a commitment to moving towards valued directions even when circumstances shift and change.

The Hadith, *"tie your camel first, and then put your trust in Allah,"* is a reminder of the importance of engagement in self-management rather than solely relying on Allah for a solution to your problems. *"Allah will not change the condition of a people until they change what is in themselves"* (Quran 13.11). Make the intention to help yourself through regular prayer and dhikr by remembering to be grateful to Allah for his mercy with Alhamdulillah (gratitude to Allah), seeking repentance by reciting Astagfirullah (seeking forgiveness), and keeping the faith by making dua to Allah. In this way, you can build a routine into your daily life and strengthen your connection with Allah.

Allah has given us the skills and resources to pursue our goals, so take appropriate measures foremost and then put your trust in Allah. For example, if your goal is to gain employment, then you can make dua that Allah increases your sustenance and makes this goal possible, but then you also need to look for jobs that fit in with your specific health needs and apply for the position. The Prophet ﷺ tells us that Allah loves actions that are consistent even if small. *"The deeds most beloved in the eyes of Allah are those deeds carried out with continuity (regularity) although they may be small"* (Sahih Muslim).

It is important in terms of pain management to consider the vicious cycle of boom and bust (over and under activity). This means on good days when the pain is more tolerable, the client may overdo some activities leading to increased pain which then reduces activity for the next day. Spend some time discussing how pacing can help break the cycle of boom and bust.

What is the boom-and-bust cycle?

For people with chronic pain, it is normal to have some good days and bad days when the pain flares up. Chronic pain often leads to people reducing physical activity because they are not able to do the same activities as they could before. This means that, when pain increases, they might either stop their activities or they might press through the pain and try to cram in as much activity as possible in case tomorrow is a bad day. Doing too much on a good day can trap us in what we call a boom-and-bust cycle which makes it much harder to manage pain and fatigue. This is when we need to be patient, pace ourselves, and gradually build up our activity levels.

If you wake up in the morning and notice that your pain is not as bad as usual and you also have a long list of jobs that you have been putting off such as cleaning, ironing, or going to the supermarket, then it may be tempting to get all the jobs done while the going is good. You decide to do as much as possible with only a few breaks to rest and feel good that you have achieved your goals. However, what happens the next morning is that the pain is worse than normal, and you barely manage to do anything. Pain medication does not help. You may even spend all day in bed recovering from the overactivity.

This leaves you out of action for a few days. In the end, the cost of overdoing the activities may be a severe flare-up of pain, irritability, lack of sleep, and lack of motivation to continue with the activities you have set for yourself. *Does this sound familiar?*

This pattern of rest and overactivity means that, over time, you may do less physical activity with an inability to endure the level of activity that you could do before. In addition, your joints and muscles may feel tense which then makes your pain worse and impacts your mood and day-to-day life. To avoid being caught up in this cycle pacing is essential.

Pacing is not about stopping activities you want to do but achieving them while maintaining an even level of activity and energy levels throughout the day. A "paced" approach gives you a way to break everyday activities and exercise into smaller bits. This means doing little bits often or finding the middle road between overdoing and underdoing. Pacing is not a sign of weakness so long as your actions are consistent. There are three overlapping elements to pacing. These include breaking tasks into small bits, taking regular breaks, and gradually increasing the amount of activity.

The client can be assisted in developing a pacing plan. The first step is to help them identify the activity that they wish to engage in from the goal they have identified.

How do I pace?

Select an activity that you enjoy and would like to do more of, for example, walking, reading the Quran, being able to play with your children, doing household chores, and visiting friends and family. It is better to start with something easier first.

A paced activity should be based on measurement (such as the amount of time, distance, and number of repetitions) rather than the amount of pain you are experiencing. Work out your starting point or a baseline, for example, how far you can walk comfortably now before the activity becomes difficult. For example, doing 15 minutes of walking or 10 minutes of light housework gives a basis from which to build "activity tolerance," which is important to allow you to do everyday tasks. Track your activity for good and bad days for at least three days to get your baseline. With this information, you can then plan for when, where, and how you will do the activity and how you can gradually build it up.

Once you start the activity, slowly increase either the time, the distance, the repetitions, or the intensity of the activity, only increasing when you feel comfortable but generally around 10% each week. It will help you to write down your progress and talk about it with someone you trust to help you keep on track and show your progress.

Remember that, by pacing, you can increase your level of activity and fitness, hence your overall sense of well-being. The gains are up to you, but keep in mind that a small amount of regular activity is better than none.

Let us look at an example of pacing. Fatima is a 42-year-old housewife. She gets lower back pain and needs to sit down a lot when the pain in her back flares up. She cannot sit for longer than 30 minutes and needs to stand up and move. Fatima feels she has drifted from family and friends as her difficulty in sitting and standing for long prevents her from visiting family and she declines invitations to weddings and gatherings as she is worried the pain might flare up and everyone will notice. As a result, she often feels despondent. Fatima would like to start visiting her elderly parents more to help them out with basic cleaning chores as she feels as their only daughter, she is neglecting her Islāmic duty towards caring for them and helping them out.

Based on her baseline, Fatima spends a couple of hours at her parent's house once a month and reasonably manages any flare-ups. Within this time, she feels she might be able to help them with some dusting and ironing. She splits the tasks up, so she does a bit at a time and rests in between. As Fatima becomes more confident, she starts to visit her parents twice a week and then eventually once a week.

Fatima feels connected with her values as she no longer feels guilty for neglecting her parents and is also managing the tasks without being caught up in a boom-and-bust situation.

Worksheet 1.4 can help the client develop their pacing plan (see Appendix 1 for the handout).

Taking regular planned relaxation breaks or planned rests even on the days when you feel good is crucial. Try to remember that, even on not-so-good days, relaxation, stretching, and short daily walks can help control the pain as avoidance of activity results in deconditioning. It is easy to drift away from faith, life, and what is important to you when living with chronic pain as you may feel stuck and unsure of what to do next, but, ultimately, it is up to you to decide the next step. You can either stay as you are or plan what to do next.

Point out that sometimes the client may find themselves relapsing into unhelpful behaviours such as avoidance or even despair. However, we can learn to understand our imperfections and use them as a chance to bring us closer to Allah. Refer to the concept of tawba to help shift the client's failure-based thoughts towards connecting with Allah.

Some people may view their chronic pain condition as a punishment from Allah for their previous misdeeds. This belief may lead to a state of apathy which may prevent them from engaging in self-management strategies because they may feel they deserve to suffer and must accept Allah's punishment. Tawba is tied with intention and at times of failure is useful to invoke as it encourages us to use prayer and patience to deal with our struggles and to maintain a sense of presence and hope. The Quranic verse "*Allah does not charge a soul except with that within its capacity*" (Holy Quran 2:286) can inspire us to keep the faith and persevere in our goals.

Worksheet 1.4 Pacing Plan

Activity	Baseline	Goal
Go for nature walks	10 minutes once a week	Increase by 5 minutes a week
Visit close family members	Once a month for an hour	To visit once a week

Tawba entails discipline and an intention of purification from past demeanours to become closer to Allah. Allah states in the Quran, *"Indeed, I am the Perpetual Forgiver of whoever repents and believes and does righteousness and then continues in guidance"* (Quran 20:82). This discussion can lead to an introduction to cognitive defusion and the benefits of cultivating present-moment awareness.

Sometimes, our plan to increase activity does not always go well. However, tripping up is an opportunity to ask Allah for help, to seek forgiveness, and to turn to him for support and guidance. The mind often slips into a negative mode when it tells us that we are not doing enough or that it is no point doing the activity if we cannot do it the way we used to or there is no point starting a new activity if we never managed to achieve it when we were well. This is often described as being in a state of cognitive fusion which is the tendency to think that our thoughts and reality are the same. When this happens, it can become hard to separate ourselves from our thoughts.

How can you fight this?

Cognitive defusion allows us to step back and detach ourselves from unhelpful thoughts, images, and memories and helps with the realisation that a thought is just a thought and nothing more. We can develop the skill to notice unhelpful thoughts and to detach from them rather than giving them power by believing in them. A metaphor that can help us take a step back from unhelpful thoughts is to think of the mind as the sky and thoughts as passing clouds.

Imagine placing your thoughts on the clouds high in the sky. Watch as the clouds slowly drift away. Remind yourself that thoughts are just like clouds and have no actual substance as they come and go.

This metaphor is a reminder that uncomfortable thoughts or feelings are fleeting, just like clouds, and do not have to be interpreted as literal truths. Remember that you are not your thoughts!

Teaching the clients how to defuse their thoughts using an Islāmic approach of attaining closeness to Allah may help validate the intervention and give people the incentive to commit to change. Remind the client that, although we are not responsible for the unintended thoughts in our minds, we should not entertain them, especially if they are unhelpful or indeed contrary to religious beliefs. Only when we deliberately decide to act on our negative thoughts, are we held accountable for them. We can learn to become more aware of thoughts, to give us the space to react appropriately, ignore what is bad, and pursue what is good.

Allah, the Merciful is aware of the state of our heart and the distress these thoughts cause the soul. No matter how good we are, we all have bad thoughts, which does not mean we are bad people for having them. To punish ourselves for having negative thoughts is destructive and counterproductive. The Prophet ﷺ said, *"Verily, Allah has pardoned my nation for their bad thoughts within themselves as long as they do not speak of them or act upon them"* (Mishkat al-Masabih 63 Book 1). This means that intention is everything.

There are many parables in the Quran about ease after hardship which can be used to help manage thoughts related to despair and helplessness. *"For indeed, with hardship will be ease"* (Quran 94.5). *"And to be firm and patient, in pain and adversity and throughout all periods of panic. Such are the people of truth, the God-fearing"* (Quran 2:177).

The Quran tells us the story of the Prophet Yusuf (Surah Yusuf), who was betrayed by his brothers and then spent years in prison, before eventually becoming the Minister of Egypt. There are many lessons that we can learn from this surah. We learn that even Prophets have been tested by Allah with trials and tribulations. Allah in his mercy has a plan for each of us even though we may find it hard to understand why we may be going through pain and suffering. Even when we do not understand what is happening to us, in hindsight, we recognize that those trials were necessary to make us a better person. We may not see the positive outcomes of our suffering in this life but know that we will be rewarded in the hereafter.

When the Prophet ﷺ and the Muslims were experiencing extreme hardship, they were reminded by Allah that difficulty is part of life, but Allah's mercy and help are also near

---

Do you think you will be admitted into Paradise without being tested like those before you? They experienced suffering and adversity and were so shaken in spirit that even the Prophet and the faithful who were with him cried, "When will Allah's help come?" Verily the help of Allah is near.

(Qur'ān 2:214)

Explain to the client that we will explore thought defusion and gratitude in more detail in the next session. Finish the session with the deep breathing exercise (see Handout 2.1, Appendix 2). Instruct the client to practice cognitive defusion by using the "clouds metaphor" to distance themselves from their thoughts.

Reference

Mishkat al-Masabih 63 Book 1, Hadith 57 https://sunnah.com/mishkat:63

9 Treatment Session 4

Agenda

- Homework review
- Cognitive defusion
- Present-moment awareness
- Self as context
- Gratitude
- Deep breathing exercise

Begin the fourth session with a review of the homework task which included the deep breathing practice and the "clouds in the sky" thought defusion exercise. Reflect on any difficulties and obstacles with the exercises. The agenda for this session is to expand on cognitive defusion to manage unhelpful thought by using present-moment awareness exercises which will also help the client to take perspective and be able to stand back and look at the limiting stories and narratives about the self objectively. The benefits of gratitude in managing mood and states of despair will also be discussed using examples from the Quran and Hadith.

Begin by describing the "leaves on a stream exercise" as another way of creating distance from unhelpful thoughts and allowing a pause between thoughts/sensations and reactions.

Leaves on a Stream

The "leaves on a stream" exercise is a gentle and calming strategy that connects us with the present moment and helps us stand back from our thoughts so that we can avoid becoming trapped by them. This exercise will help you distance yourself from your thoughts so that, instead of seeing the world from inside your thoughts, you will view your thoughts from afar from a more objective stance.

DOI:10.4324/9781003329626-11

Find a comfortable position and imagine you are sitting by the side of a gently flowing stream, with leaves floating past on the surface of that stream. Imagine the sounds of water gently flowing over the rocks. Whenever a thought enters your mind, briefly observe it, place it upon a leaf, and watch as it floats down the stream. Do this with every thought that pops into your head, regardless of the type of thought whether good or bad, pleasant, or painful. If your thoughts stop or the leaf gets stuck, that is fine. Allow it to hang around or pause and continue to watch the stream. Just allow the stream to flow at its speed.

If you start thinking, this is silly, or I cannot do this, place those thoughts on a leaf ("I am now thinking this is silly"). If you notice a difficult feeling arising such as impatience or frustration, simply acknowledge it. Saying to yourself, "I have a feeling of frustration" or "I notice a feeling of impatience." Then place those words on a leaf and let them float away.

From time to time, your thoughts will take over and you might lose track of the exercise. This is expected and will happen. As soon as you notice your thoughts beginning to wander, gently acknowledge them and then start the exercise again.

Spend around five minutes on this exercise. Once the exercise has been completed, ask the client to think about the following questions:

What sort of thoughts distracted your mind?
What was it like to let thoughts come and go without becoming caught up in them?
Was it hard to let go of any thoughts in particular? For example, any positive thoughts?
Did any feelings show up? If they did then just acknowledge them again as you did in the exercise

The aforementioned questions will elicit any difficulties that the client may experience with present-moment awareness and thought defusion. Use this opportunity to explain how we all tend to over-identify with our thoughts, by strengthening them in our minds as "facts and truths."

By using cognitive defusion to notice thoughts rather than becoming caught up in them, we become aware of the actual process of our thinking, and this can reduce the influence of thoughts on our behaviours and increase our ability to be present and take effective action.

Remind the client that, with regular practice, the leaves on a stream exercise will become easier and have powerful positive effects to help them distance themselves from negative internal experiences without needing to struggle with them.

Another way of helping the client to create cognitive defusion or space from unhelpful thoughts is present-moment awareness which helps us to exercise our mind to create resilience just as physical training exercises the body and increases health and well-being.

Practising present-moment awareness can help us develop a state of mind that can enhance the quality of our obligatory acts of worship as we are more likely to be able to perform the daily salah with presence knowing that a beautiful conversation is taking place with Allah during the salah. In this way, our awareness of Allah as being omnipresent will strengthen.

In terms of chronic pain, negative or worrisome thoughts whether related to physical sensations or otherwise can affect mood and increase the perception of pain. The practice of contemplation can assist in separating thoughts from the self to allow us to concentrate on relaxing the body, observing the breath and bodily sensations simply as they are. This helps reduce pain perception as well as reduce the symptoms of depression and anxiety.

When pain sensations worsen, instead of ignoring them or distracting from them, mindfully addressing the characteristics of these sensations can allow us to step back from the pain, make room for other feelings, and make more accurate appraisals.

An exercise that can help cultivate present-moment awareness of pain is to locate the part of your body that is giving you the greatest pain and focus on that area. Identify whether the discomfort is neutral, mild, or heavy. Does it feel hot, cold, or neutral? Is the pain moving or is it static? Does it feel solid, or is it dispersed? Rather than repressing sensations and emotions, holding awareness of the body and emotions can allow us to get used to the sensations instead of fighting or reacting emotionally to them. It is then possible to develop gradual acceptance and the willingness to accept that Allah is the one who governs health and disease and is the ultimate healer.

Being present in the moment is often considered to be a modern psychological tool, but it is a practice rooted in Islāmic belief as we are compelled to seek Allah mindfully in every action as a form of worship. Being in a state of present-moment awareness allows us to become conscious of Allah and our relationship with Him with the knowledge that Allah is fully aware of our every deed and action. When we become heedless, we pay too much unnecessary attention to the world which weakens our ability to remain in the present and reduces tawakkul.

There are other less formal ways in which present-moment awareness can be practised as a way of connecting with Allah. One of these is to go for mindful walks which means paying attention to your surroundings and the environment and using your senses to live in the moment instead of walking while on autopilot with a mind overrun with unhelpful thought processes. Just noticing the trees, the colours of the leaves, the flowers and the different varieties, the environment, and so forth allows us to feel in awe of Allah's creations invoking Alhamdulillah.

Being present can be practiced while showering or performing wudhu (ritual ablutions). Just pay attention to the way the water falls on your skin, the way the lather of the soap spreads across your skin, and the sensation it creates, and at each step, remain focussed on your actions rather than your thoughts even though you may be aware of them.

While praying salah, focus on the recitation and each ritual movement while being mindful that you are in the presence of Allah Almighty and in conversation with Him. Recite the verses with purpose and meaning and every time your mind wanders gently bring it back to the present by remembering you have an audience with your Lord.

Daily exercises that complement the obligatory acts of worship are to engage in dhikr and make supplications. Dhikr has been shown to increase the secretion of endorphins to induce a feeling of well-being and comfort. For this reason, chronic pain sufferers who practice constant dhikr with each heartbeat and breath can train their minds, hearts, and bodies to cultivate peace, wellness, and contentment: "*Surely in the remembrance of Allah do hearts find comfort. Those who believe and do good, for them will be bliss and an honourable destination*" (Quran 13:28–29).

Using dhikr and prayer as a means of increasing our proximity to Allah can help us learn to overcome the distress of unwanted thoughts and sensations and to remain grounded in the present moment rather than becoming caught in a state of mental time travel, lamenting over past mistakes, or worrying about the future.

It may help to remember that Allah has taken the past and the future out of our hands. All the regrets of the past cannot be undone but are lessons to be learnt. The future is also in Allah's hands as even though we make plans "*Not even a leaf falls without His (Allah's) knowledge*" (Quran 6:59). You only have the responsibility for the present which should be enjoyed as a gift. Use the present time to increase your connection with Allah and cultivate a quality of life aligned with your values. With intention and presence, we can develop accountability and awareness and learn to control our wandering minds and discipline our thoughts. "*Verily in the remembrance of Allah, there is contentment of the heart*" (Quran 13:28).

At times of emotional or physical difficulty, reciting dhikr using the tasbih beads can help us connect with Allah and anchor us into the state of being present. This exercise is a useful way of helping you not only to defuse unhelpful thoughts but also to nourish the heart and mind and increase your spiritual connection to the Creator. "*Be mindful of Allah and Allah will protect you. Be mindful of Allah and you will find him in front of you*" (Hadith an Nawawi 40:19).

The "Dropping Anchor" exercise helps to bring us back to the present moment and can metaphorically help us observe the storm of life without being caught up in it, just like a boat would anchor itself when caught in the middle of a storm. Dhikr remembrance can function as an "anchor" to ground us in the here and now. An anchor in this context is a soothing phrase that the mind will learn to associate with the state of being present and can be used not only while practicing a formal grounding exercise but also at other times when unhelpful thoughts become overwhelming.

An anchor using the tasbih dhikr could be any one of the glorious names of Allah or any other supplications from the Sunnah for example it has been narrated that "*two words are beloved to the Most Merciful, light on the tongue but heavy on the scale: Glory and praise to Allah (Subhan Allah wa bihamdihi), and glory to Allah Almighty (Subhan Allahil Athim)*" (Sahih al-Bukhari 7563). And "*The best remembrance is to declare there is no God but Allah (la ilhaha illa Allah), and the best supplication is to declare all praise is due to Allah (Al-hamdulillah)*" (Jami` at-Tirmidhi 3383). The Prophet ﷺ used "*istighfar*" (seeking forgiveness of Allah) regularly as one of his anchors.

Present-Moment Awareness Exercise Using Tasbih Dhikr

Let us begin the exercise with you choosing an anchor. Next, focus your awareness on your breathing and start to take slow breaths just like you have learnt with the weekly breathing exercise. You can either close your eyes or focus on a point on the floor. Scan your body and try to relax any area of your body where there may be muscle tension. With each breath, gauge the state of your heart and mind for any thoughts, feelings, or sensations, and then bring back the awareness to your breath. Take each breath with gratitude to Allah for the life and energy he has given you. Start to anchor your thoughts and roll each bead through your fingers. Be mindful of the texture of the bead while focusing on the recitation you are making. Every time your mind wanders, return your attention to Allah with an awareness of His watchful presence. Just focus on your chosen recitation while continuing to roll the tasbih beads through your fingers.

Think of your mind as if it were a still pond and your thoughts are ripples and waves in this pond. Be aware of the ripples but remember you can also choose to ignore them as engaging in them will only make the waves stronger. Notice the waves and ripples, acknowledge them, and allow them to simply disperse while you anchor yourself and return your attention to the here and now.

Continue this practice for at least five minutes . . .

The repeated practice will help the mind associate these recitations with the presence of the heart connected to Allah and will strengthen the ability to remain grounded in the here and now, in Allah's remembrance with the knowledge that He is always with you.

Remember that even when you are present before Allah, the mind will wander off and become distracted by emerging thoughts. Present-moment awareness in this context is not about silencing our thoughts, but simply becoming aware of them and learning to let them pass. The more conscious we are of our thoughts, the more distance we can create between ourselves and them. Only then can we stop becoming our thoughts.

With continued practice, you will strengthen your mental and spiritual ability to be able to diffuse from these thoughts and remain present in the moment. This may take time but the more you repeat the exercise while in a state of gratitude for Allah's mercy and blessings, the easier it will become to put a distance between unhelpful thought processes and reactivity.

Explain to the client that being present in their mind can help them become more aware of their thinking patterns and the problematic stories they tell themselves. This can help them become aware of the self as context rather than the self as content and create distance from their self-stories, preventing them from becoming trapped in them.

The thoughts, feelings, stories, and judgements that you have about yourself are a part of you, but they are not the whole of you. You are much more than these. It is important to develop an awareness of your internal processes in order not to be dictated by misleading self-stories. This will help you cultivate a state of mind where the realities of both mental and emotional states become clearer without you becoming entrapped with your thoughts and internal sensations and as such can help to control the nafs or ego.

By being in a state of presence, we can free ourselves from being attached to erroneous self-stories or limiting beliefs and develop the resilience to stand back and see things as they are. For example, instead of defining yourself as "useless," you may change your perspective to "*I may feel useless sometimes, but I am not useless.*" Change the commentary of your mind from being in the experience to observing the experience. Just like a commentator of a football match who describes what is happening in the football game but is not experiencing the game. This will help you defuse these experiences and make room for seeing thoughts and feelings for what they are and help you anchor yourself and find safety within. While you are practicing any present-moment awareness exercise whether it be breathing, body scan, walking, leaves on a stream, dhikr, and so on, notice the pain, thought, feeling, and sensation, and become aware that you are noticing that there is a part of you observing your private experiences and giving a commentary on what is happening.

Introduce the concept of gratitude as a way of overcoming feelings of despair. Briefly explain how neuroscience has shown that gratitude can help, increase resilience, well-being, and social relationships, and reduce symptoms of depression and anxiety (Korb, 2015) and the importance of gratitude in Islām.

When we are experiencing challenging times in our life, it is easy to descend into a state of helplessness and often despair and question our fate while seeing every difficulty as a catastrophe. At these times, showing gratitude can be an antidote. Gratitude may not always be easy to practice when we are overwhelmed by pain or emotional difficulties, and it may feel jarring to be told to be grateful or that we have so much to be grateful for. However, remember that, while gratitude does not change our situation, it can help us shift focus to make the situation less overwhelming.

Research tells us that feelings of gratitude stimulate the production of dopamine in the brain which is the feel-good neurotransmitter that plays a role in increasing well-being and motivation and can reduce symptoms of anxiety and depression (Liang et al 2020). Allah also tells us about the importance of gratitude: "*remember Me; I will remember you. And thank Me, and never be ungrateful*" (Quran 2:152) and "*if you are grateful, I will give you more of my blessings*" (Quran 14:7).

As humans any hardship may seem far from desirable but enduring it with gratitude during tough times can help transform the burden of pain and help us develop a perspective beyond the distress of the moment, making the trial of suffering easier to bear (Abdi, 2014). The

Quran reminds us: *"You may dislike something although it is good for you, or like something although it is bad for you: God knows, and you do not"* (Quran 2: 216).

The humble dandelion plant is believed to be an inconvenient weed in the garden, yet for thousands of years, herbalists have used it as a medicinal plant because it is packed with nutrients and is effective in detoxifying the blood. Likewise, every trouble in our life may be a great inconvenience, but, if faced with patience and gratitude, it is likely to be a gift sent to strengthen our character and increase resilience. Gratitude is not a passive process. The more gratitude we cultivate, the deeper it resides in the heart and the more resilience we develop to face our challenges.

Allah with his grace and perfection has wired our brains to create happiness whilst in obeyance to Him which is why regardless of our spiritual state when we are tested with difficulties such as physical illness, pain, or emotional distress and loss, our first reaction is to turn to Allah for help. Difficult though it may be to comprehend, the purpose of hardship is so that we can return to Allah.

Contemplation upon the blessings of Allah is not only a form of meditation, but it is worship and creates contentment and acceptance regardless of the difficulties you may be facing. By showing gratitude to the Almighty, hope and trust in Allah's plan becomes stronger we are more likely to become aware of the positives in our life and opportunities.

Maintaining a state of remembrance in the Almighty, with gratitude for Allah's mercy and blessings, is a means of becoming more mindful of His presence and the importance of living a life in preparation for the hereafter. *"God always rewards gratitude and He knows everything"* (Quran, 4:147). The importance of gratitude is that it is not beneficial for others but for our souls. *"Be grateful to Allah for whoso is grateful is grateful for the good of his own soul"* (Quran 31:12).

The first lesson on gratitude can be seen in Surah Fatiha which is the starting chapter of the Quran and begins with the word Alhamdulillah. The essence of Alhamdulillah is "All praise is for Allah," with the belief that no matter what the circumstances are, whether we are in pain, sorrow, sickness, or fear, Allah knows what is best for us.

The first lesson on gratitude can be seen in Surah Fatiha which is the starting chapter of the Quran and begins with the word Alhamdulillah. The essence of Alhamdulillah is "All praise is for Allah," with the belief that no matter what the circumstances are, whether we are in pain, sorrow, sickness, or fear, Allah knows what is best for us.

Cultivate gratitude as an attitude towards life because with it we can neutralize the negative emotions related to our Nafs (ego), such as jealousy, arrogance, resentment, low self-esteem, lack of motivation, and laziness, amongst many other emotions. Being in a state of gratitude helps to polish the soul from such negative feelings. No matter how long your mind has been spent in a state of heedlessness, every time you bring it back to Allah's remembrance with silent gratitude for your life and breath, the easier it will become.

Ask yourself; are you not still alive despite your difficulties? Do you still see the sun rising, the birds singing, and the flowers blooming? Do you still have the comfort of a roof over your head, and food on the table with the blessings of family and community? If the answer is yes to even one of those questions, then it is a reminder that Allah is not punishing you but prompting you to look at the many blessings that are taken for granted. When all ends, we can be reminded by the Quran that Allah loves us because He is *"closer to you than your jugular vein"* (Quran 50:16). We can remind ourselves that *"Verily, with the hardship, there is relief"* (Quran 95:5) and those who endure trials and tribulations in life will be rewarded in the hereafter. *"Whenever a Muslim is afflicted by harm from sickness or other matters, God will expiate his sins, like leaves drop from a tree"* (Sahih al-Bukhari 5647).

End the session with the deep breathing exercise (see Appendix 2). Reiterate the homework exercises and provide the client with Handouts 2.3, 2.4, and 2.5 (Appendix 2) to practice until the next session. Remind the client that dhikr can be practiced after Salah, preferably after the dawn (fajr) prayer or at least at a regular time daily. The client can spend as much time as they wish on dhikr, but at the very least, they should devote at least five minutes every day to help consolidate their practice and make it a long-term habit.

References

Hadith 19, 40 Hadith an Nawawi. https://sunnah.com/nawawi40:19.

Ambara Abdi Gratitude in Times of Hardship Published April 11, 2014. https://messageinternational.org/gratitude-in-times-of-hardship/

Korb, A. (2015). *Upward spiral: Using neuroscience to reverse the course of depression, one small change at a time*. New Harbinger.

Liang, H., Chen, C., Li, F. et al. Mediating effects of peace of mind and rumination on the relationship between gratitude and depression among Chinese university students. Curr Psychol 39, 1430–1437 (2020). https://doi.org/10.1007/s12144-018-9847-1

Jami` at-Tirmidhi 3383, Book 48, Hadith 14, Vol. 6, Book 45. https://sunnah.com/tirmidhi/48/14

Riyad as-Salihin 1408 , Book 15, Hadith 1. https://sunnah.com/riyadussalihin:1408

Sahih al-Bukhari 7563 Book 97, Hadith 188. https://sunnah.com/bukhari:7563

Sahih al-Bukhari 5647 Book 75, Hadith 7. https://sunnah.com/bukhari:5647

10 Treatment Session 5

Agenda

- Homework review
- Mood management
- Sleep hygiene
- Relaxation exercise

In this session, spend around 5–10 minutes discussing the homework activities and whether the client felt able to engage in the dhikr and gratitude exercises. It is not unusual for clients to struggle with these exercises as they are likely to be new to them. Remind the client that patience and perseverance are the key when starting to incorporate new habits.

This session will explore how the complex experience of chronic pain can increase the risk of depression, anxiety, and other mental health issues.

Even though there are a variety of reasons behind this correlation including lack of acceptance, loss of identity, and pain catastrophising, a recent study reported in the European Journal of Pain (Kang et al., 2021) highlighted the connection between chronic pain and mental health conditions. The researchers found that people with chronic pain have an imbalance of certain chemical messengers in the brain that are responsible for regulating emotions.

Providing the client with a scientific rationale for the link between chronic pain and low mood and depression can be helpful to get the client on board with self-management and help those struggling with pain to understand that the depression or anxiety they may be experiencing is linked to brain changes that come from persistent pain. This helps to contextualise their symptoms and provide a better understanding of the importance of mood management thereby increasing compliance.

Many a time in our day-to-day lives, we face physical and emotional demands that become overwhelming and almost impossible to manage. For chronic pain sufferers, it becomes a vicious cycle of pain and

DOI:10.4324/9781003329626-12

emotional distress such as feelings of depression, anxiety, anger, frustration, and despair which perpetuate one another.

Research tells us that there is a link between chronic pain and mental health conditions due to a chemical imbalance that occurs when people have persistent pain. The cycle of chronic pain and the perpetual discomfort with modified activity in the brain can impact our mood state and other areas of physical health, such as sleep, memory, concentration, and appetite. This can make it difficult to function at work or at home or participate in enjoyable activities which is why it is important to address these factors.

Depression and anxiety can often be a response to the challenges of living with chronic pain especially when left untreated or when all hope of it being eliminated is removed. These feelings worsen when we have certain expectations about how we want to live our life. When our realities do not match our hopes, this can create a sense of hopelessness and maladaptive thinking patterns. These emotions interfere with our ability to experience a true connection to Allah, and even though we may be aware of Allah's love and mercy, we may start believing that sadness is a sign of weak faith and descend into the distorted belief that Allah has left us or chosen not to bless us.

There are several lessons we can take from the Quran to help us navigate our emotional responses to chronic pain and distress. Sura ad-Duha (Quran 93:1–8) was revealed to the Prophet Muhammed ﷺ at a time when he was going through a period of trials and tribulations and felt depressed and anxious thinking that Allah had forsaken him. This surah gave the Prophet ﷺ the reassurance, strength, and resilience to face his difficulties. If we allow ourselves to ponder on the example of the best of creation and how he managed his distress, then we can also create the impetus to manage challenges in our own life.

The verse *"Your Lord has neither forsaken you nor has He become displeased"* (Quran 93:3) powerfully emphasises the concept of attachment and the need to feel we have someone at times of hardship. Allah tells us that He does not hate us and has not forgotten us which is a reminder that He is always present. *"And if you come to Me walking, I will come to you running"* (Hadith Qudsi 15).

Often at times of difficulty or elevated pain and distress, our faith may waver with a decline in our spiritual connection with Allah especially if we feel like our prayers are not being answered, or that our dhikr/worship is not having a positive impact on our well-being. We may have questions such as *"Is this how my life is going to be? Is it ever going to become better? Am I being punished for my sins?"*

Reflecting on the above Surah can help foster hope, positivity, and reassurance in its reminder that, after darkness, there is light and that things will not always be the same. With every sunrise, there is an opportunity for goodness, growth, and change, so we should look forward to that which is yet to come.

By the Glorious Morning Light, and by the Night when it is still, your Lord has neither forsaken you nor has He become displeased. And surely the hereafter will be better for you than the present (life). And soon your lord will grant you, and you shall be well-pleased.

(Quran 93:1–5)

The aforementioned verses remind us that life in this world is temporary, and our permanent abode will be the hereafter, a place for us to look forward to. When we feel despairing, by turning to Allah's promise to provide something better, we can strengthen our resilience to overcome pain and become steadfast in our faith and motivation.

The practice of gratitude daily has been shown to relieve us of physical and psychological symptoms. Gratitude does not change our situation, but, as discussed in the previous session, it is a powerful way to overcome negative feelings about the situation as it helps us shift focus. People who are experiencing difficulties with physical and mental health often feel that nobody could be in a worse situation than they are. Sura ad-Duha refers to the importance of gratitude with the verses *"So as for the orphan, do not oppress [him]. And as for the petitioner, do not repel [him]. But as for the favour of your Lord, report [it]"* (Quran 93:9–11).

This verse is a reminder that there are people in far worse situations (orphans and beggars). We should remember them to overcome our distress and reconnect with Allah, in open gratitude for the many gifts He has bestowed upon us. If Allah can turn night into day, he can without doubt relieve the burden of physical and psychological distress for those who turn to Him. Therefore, remembrance with gratitude for Allah's mercy and blessings serves to bring ease from trials as stated in the following verse of the Quran:

"We certainly know that your heart is truly distressed by what they say. So, glorify the praises of your Lord and be one of those who always pray, and worship your Lord until the inevitable comes your way" (Quran 15:97–99). The Quran is constantly telling us not to give up hope and turn to worship in times of difficulty.

When discussing poor mental health with clients, it is also important to address how people with chronic pain tend to experience disrupted sleep patterns which can worsen their mental state.

There is often a vicious cycle between sleep disruption and pain. It is often hard to determine whether the pain is causing the sleep problems, or whether poor quality sleep is exacerbating the pain. For example, pain symptoms may be the main reason that you wake at night with disrupted sleep and reduced quality of restful sleep. Unfortunately, continuous sleep deprivation can lower our pain threshold and our tolerance for pain causing the pain to feel intolerable.

Sleep is essential for good physical and mental health as it provides rest so that the body can recuperate and restore itself. Sleep is mentioned repeatedly in the Quran. *"And among his signs is your sleep by night and by day and your seeking of His bounty, verily in that are Signs for those who listen"* (Quran 30:23). There is no doubt that sleep is a mercy from Allah, and the aforementioned verse emphasises the benefits of keeping to a pattern of light and darkness. The verse in Sura ad-Duha *"and the night when it falls still!"* (Quran 93:2) refers to the night as a time of stillness suggesting comfort and rest

Modern science has identified sleep stages and sleep hygiene rules that correspond with those recommended in Islām. Research has found that a regular light–dark cycle is essential for maintaining the circadian rhythms that control bodily functioning and hormone release (David, 2009). The Prophet Muhammed ﷺ said, *"Put out lamps when you go to bed, shut the doors, and cover water and food containers"* (Sahih Bukhari 5301) which corresponds with the findings on the importance of a dark environment when trying to induce sleep.

Furthermore, the quality of sleep can be significantly disturbed by noise because it causes more arousal and more changes in the stages of sleep and disrupts the rhythms of rapid eye movement (REM) which is important for stimulating the areas of the brain that are important for learning and memory (Muzet, 2007). This is why poor sleep often makes people feel they have "brain fog." Chronic sleep disturbance has also been linked to an increase in the risk of cardiovascular disease (Goines & Hagler, 2007).

The Quran mentions in Sura Al-Kahf the importance of noise minimisation to help create a suitable environment for sleep while referring to the "sleepers in the cave." The hearing of the sleepers was sealed during the entire period they spent in the cave. *"Therefore, We covered up their (sense of) hearing (causing them to go in deep sleep) in the Cave for a number of years"* (Quran 18:11).

A good sleep hygiene pattern would entail creating a quiet and soothing environment and sleeping in a darkened room to induce relaxation and sleep.

Many chronic pain sufferers may sleep during the day because of a lack of sleep at night. Studies in neuroscience demonstrate that taking a nap during the day improves memory, alertness, performance, and some aspects of lost nighttime sleep (Tumiran et al., 2018). Midday napping (referred to as Qailulah) was also a practice recommended by Prophet Muhammed ﷺ. The Prophet ﷺ said, "*Sleeping early in the day betrays ignorance, in the middle of the day is right, and at the end of the day is stupid*" (Bahamman, 2011). Another Hadith reported, "*We used to offer the Jumma (Friday) prayer with the Prophet and then take the afternoon nap*" (Sahih Bukhri 941).

The best way to benefit from a short nap is to limit it to 30 minutes in the afternoon. However, given that many people with chronic pain experience fatigue, they may be tempted to sleep for longer periods. It is important to explain to the client that taking excessively long daytime naps is counterproductive and will disrupt the internal body clock and perpetuate sleep disorders. If a client cannot limit their daytime nap to a maximum of an hour, then it is not advisable nor is sleeping in the late afternoon recommended.

Some people may find daytime napping difficult due to pain, but just taking some time to rest and relax in the early afternoon can also provide benefits. This can be achieved by creating a restful environment, by being in a quiet, dark place with a comfortable room temperature and without distractions.

However, when recommending sleep hygiene strategies to chronic pain clients, it is important to remain mindful that there are diagnosis-specific characteristics found in different chronic pain conditions. For example, people with conditions such as fibromyalgia or complex regional pain syndrome tend to have a higher sensory sensitivity and report excessive fatigue and insomnia compared to other pain conditions. The effectiveness of sleep hygiene methods for this population is likely to be impacted by this. It may be necessary to tailor any sleep hygiene strategies to take these factors into account.

Poor sleep habits, such as napping for extended hours during the day, excessive caffeine intake, and staying up late watching TV or using other electronic devices can cause and worsen sleep difficulties. Using an ACT approach to managing sleep entails any relaxing activities that fit in with the client's lifestyle and work for them. For example, avoiding the use of a mobile phone or other electric devices before bed is a common sleep hygiene strategy, but, for some chronic pain clients, it may be a way of distracting from the pain symptoms.

Rather than distraction, the client is encouraged to focus on being more mindful by lying in bed with a non-judgemental acceptance of the present moment despite the discomfort. Remind the client that the goal is to reduce any negative associations with sleep time and reduce arousal levels to create a more healthy and flexible approach to sleep.

When we struggle to sleep whether it be due to physical discomfort or emotional overwhelm, our thoughts take over and create worry which then can make it more difficult to fall asleep. Pre-bedtime activities that are likely to help include using relaxation techniques, deep breathing exercises that allow mindful awareness and acceptance of internal sensations, using positive calming associations with the bedroom, and letting the body rest rather than forcing sleep.

By using present-moment awareness, we can learn to notice our senses and emotions and take them for what they are. We can defuse them by standing back to observe our level of wakefulness or unwanted thoughts and emotional reactions without becoming trapped in the sensations we might be experiencing. When we start defusing our thoughts, we learn that these thoughts don't have the power to stop us from sleeping, unless we give them that power by becoming caught up in them.

When the mind becomes overwhelmed with unhelpful thoughts. First identify, describe, and name the negative thoughts you are having about not being able to sleep. Try to identify emotions and physical sensations by objectively locating and describing the emotions or physical feelings and imagining them as objects and giving them a physical shape and colour just like in the exercise we did in our previous session.

To do this, locate the part of your body that is giving you the greatest pain and focus on that area. Identify whether the discomfort is neutral, mild, or heavy. Does it feel hot, cold, or neutral? Is the pain moving or is it static? Does it feel solid, or is it dispersed? This exercise can allow a gradual acceptance and willingness to accept the discomfort without struggling against it. Remind yourself that Allah is the healer. While doing this exercise, try reciting Allah's name Ya Shafi as a form of dhikr.

If the overwhelm is intense use the grounding exercise by noticing five things that you can see, four things you can hear, three things you can feel, two things you can touch, and one thing you can taste to calm your nervous system and bring you to the present moment. Simply being present without worrying about the past or future or somewhere else can help take the focus away from the pain and discomfort.

Other valued sleep-inducing strategies that we can use include listening to Quranic recitations, dhikr, making positive calming associations with the bedroom, and focusing on resting rather than sleep. Even when we struggle to sleep remember that our body and mind can still get rest while lying in bed, and this can take the pressure off the urgency to sleep and allow us to relax.

Teaching the client relaxation is important as chronic pain can lead to a perpetual state of body tension which then increases the perception of pain. The client can be taught the two following exercises to practice in their own time to manage pain and emotions.

Relaxation Exercise

Stress and tension in the body can make the pain worse and vice versa. Relaxation techniques can help induce sleep and manage pain.

To start this exercise, find a comfortable place to sit or lie down and make sure you will not be disturbed. Close your eyes and start by focusing on your breathing. Just as we have practiced deep breathing at each session, get yourself comfortable and breathe deeply for a few minutes. With each out-breath, release any tension in your body and allow your limbs to become limp. Continue breathing mindfully and then start to scan your body and become aware of any sensations in your body. If you notice any discomfort or sensations, direct your attention to that part of your body and breathe into that area while allowing the sensations to happen. Pay attention to any changes of intensity to those sensations. Notice any areas of your body that have a greater intensity and describe them.

What colour is the sensation? Does it have a shape? Can you make a visual image of that sensation? Does it feel hot or cold? At the same time, continue to breathe deeply and know you are in control.

Now think about how you might change the colour, shape, and temperature of the sensation so that it feels more comfortable. Could you shrink it and soften it? or make it a lighter colour or a more calming colour? What about the temperature? Does it feel better turned up or turned down? Start with some small subtle changes to the sensation.

Continue breathing in and out while making changes to the sensations until you begin to feel the discomfort bearable. As you start to feel more relaxed, use your imagination to take your mind to a place where you feel calm, happy, and safe. It can be anywhere whether it is in the countryside, near the beach, in a place of prayer whether at home, or in a nurturing person's home. Anywhere that feels calming and relaxing. Stay there for a few minutes.

Now pay attention to your breathing again and with each breath notice that you are feeling lighter and more alert and more mindful of your surroundings and gradually return your focus to the room you are sitting in. Take four more breaths, and each time you take a breath, notice you are more alert. As you finish this exercise, open your eyes and gently stretch your body.

Once the client has completed this exercise, ask them for feedback and address any concerns and doubts. If the client is not convinced of the usefulness of this for increasing pain tolerance and helping sleep, remind them that this exercise will be more effective when practised regularly and will need a commitment from them to practice daily to notice any benefits.

Move on to teaching the client the shorter body scan exercise and explain that this can be used to identify any areas of tension in the body and to be able to actively release tension.

Sometimes, a short body scan might be preferred to induce relaxation. In this case, the following body scan can be done. If practiced regularly, it can be used anywhere (Handout 2.7, Appendix 2).

Short Body Scan Exercise

If you notice any tension in your body or feel the stress levels rising, take a deep breath (as practised previously) and keep breathing slowly and deeply for a few minutes. Let your shoulders droop and relax your hands. As you continue to take slow, deep breaths starting from your feet, tense and relax the muscles before moving upwards from your feet to your legs, thighs, hips, stomach, hands, arms, chest, shoulders, neck, and then your face and head. As you focus on each area of your body, tense that part, hold for a few seconds, and then let go of the tension and notice the difference. This will enable you to become more conscious of how your body feels both when it is tense and when it is relaxed. Try to practise it as often as possible but at least once a day if you can. Over time, you will be able to do a body scan anytime, anyplace whether you are sitting down or standing, at home or even in crowded places, and release tension from your body (Handout 2.8).

Bring the session to an end, and as the client has already practiced breathing with the relaxation exercise, the deep breathing exercise can be omitted. Inform the client that the next session will be the last and will be a recap of the previous sessions and a maintenance plan will be discussed. For homework, give the client relaxation and body scan exercises to practice (Handouts 2.6 and 2.7, Appendix 2). In preparation for the end of the therapeutic sessions, ask the client to carry out a reflection practice over the next week to assess their progress and what changes they feel they have been able to implement (any committed actions), especially in terms of the spiritual aspects of the therapeutic intervention and what problems they may have encountered.

References

Bahammam, A. S. (2011). Sleep from an Islamic perspective. *Annals of Thoracic Medicine, 6*(4), 187–192. https://doi.org/10.4103/1817-1737.84771

David, R. (2009). Circadian rhythms: Calibrating the clock. *Nature Reviews Molecular Cell Biology, 10*, 816.

Goines, L., & Hagler, L. (2007). Noise pollution: A modem plague. *Southern Medical Journal, 100*, 287–294.

Hadith 15, 40 Hadith Qudsi https://sunnah.com/qudsi40:15

Kang, D., Hesam-Shariati, N., McAuley, J. H., Alam, M., Trost, Z., Rae, C. D., & Gustin, S. M. (2021). Disruption to normal excitatory and inhibitory function within the medial prefrontal cortex in people with chronic pain. *European Journal of Pain*. Published online July 9, 2021. https://doi.org/10.1002/ejp.1838

Muzet, A. (2007). Environmental noise, sleep, and health. *Sleep Medicine Reviews, 11*, 135–142.

Sahih al-Bukhari 941, Book 11, Hadith 65 https://sunnah.com/bukhari:941

Tumiran, M. A., Rahman, N. N. A., Saat, R. M., Kabir, N., Zulkifli, M. Y., & Adli, D. S. H. (2018). The Concept of Qailulah (Midday Napping) from neuroscientific and Islamic perspectives. *Journal of Religion and Health, 57*(4), 1363–1375. https://doi.org/10.1007/s10943-015-0093-7

11 Treatment Session 6

Agenda

- Homework review
- Review of previous sessions
- Spiritual growth and resilience
- Maintenance plan

Begin with a review of the previous session and the homework tasks. The client will be reminded that this is the last session. Explore how they have found the therapy sessions and their progress in being able to implement any of the strategies (any committed actions) and any obstacles to them applying the processes of ACT to their life. Check for their progress related to the spiritual aspects of the therapeutic intervention, whether it has helped them manage pain and emotions more effectively, and what might help improve this.

Remind the client that the therapy sessions are only a start to their journey of pain management as all the processes that have been covered need to be integrated into the client's daily life and practised regularly. The agenda will include summarising some of the topics we have covered thus far, guidelines for maintaining spiritual growth, and a maintenance plan for the client to continue their progress in managing chronic pain.

> Over the last few sessions, we have covered a variety of strategies aimed at helping you develop the resilience to cope effectively with the challenges of pain and illness. In the first session, we talked about how living with chronic pain can lead to unhelpful behavioural changes in people due to their fear of aggravating pain. These include avoidance behaviours that may impact work, relationships, and spirituality. The natural response to aversive situations is to avoid them, and while sometimes it may be adaptive, it is harmful when we pull away from valued activities.

DOI:10.4324/9781003329626-13

Encourage the client to focus on cultivating a healthier form of acceptance in which they neither succumb to their condition nor focus on eradication but instead are active and responsive and develop different behaviour patterns and habits to adjust to the different demands of persistent pain without compromising their values.

> We reflected on the success and failure of some of these strategies to manage pain and identified that engaging in experiential avoidance is not only a short-term solution but can intensify the experience we are avoiding leading to a cycle of psychological suffering. We discussed your willingness to acknowledge, allow (tolerate), and eventually accept reality as it is and worked towards identifying valued activities in order to reduce the struggle with pain and learn acceptance.

Passive acceptance may create more harm than good and can lead to the client slipping into adopting the "sick role" instead of improving self-efficacy. This point can be illustrated by referring back to the *"tie your camel"* hadith.

> Many people with chronic pain question the fairness of their suffering and may feel they have been abandoned by Allah. Others may feel their chronic pain is a punishment for their past deeds. Furthermore, the medical journey to finding a cure and treatment for chronic pain can be harrowing with many pain patients feeling that the health system has failed them. These thoughts and feelings can cause considerable distress and create "why me" responses that can elevate distress.
>
> It is important to remember that sadness, helplessness, and hopelessness are common reactions to living with physical and mental health difficulties and are the metaphoric "unwanted/uninvited guests." Just like we discussed when using the Guest House poem and the cactus metaphor, we cannot always remove the source of pain and difficulty, but, by pivoting towards acceptance of difficult conditions, it is possible to overcome the discomfort of these undesired internal experiences. Remember these internal events are transient, and by dropping the fear of these experiences, it is possible to remain aware of them without struggle and resistance.
>
> By acknowledging and accepting the difficulties of living with chronic pain while also actively pursuing meaning and purpose in life and taking control where it is possible, we can develop a healthy relationship with our body, with others, and with Allah Almighty.

Revisit the goals they have identified and encourage them to remain committed to them.

Clarifying values helps us pay attention to the things that are truly important, and once we realise that the pain condition has been distracting us from these important activities, we can choose to make a commitment towards change that is aligned with our personal and religious values to help break out of the "stuckness" or vicious circle of chronic pain. **How many times have you tried to avoid an activity because you thought the pain would get in the way?**

If you recall a time when this happened and someone forced you to engage in an activity you were avoiding, you will realise that it helped you remove your focus from the pain to enjoying the moment. This is why setting goals and making a commitment to act on them is important as not only does it break you out of the vicious cycle of pain, but it also helps you find a life beyond pain. It means you can start to learn to live with pain rather than against it. Acceptance of chronic pain or other life's tribulations is difficult; however, Islām has taught us that even when in the depth of despair, practising patience, gratitude, and a willingness to act on our values can help purify our soul and strengthen our ability to cope. *"Oh, you who believe! Seek help with patient perseverance and prayer, for God is with those who patiently persevere"* (Quran 2:153).

Reiterate the concept of using sabr and tawakkul during times of difficulty.

We discussed the concepts of sabr (patience) and tawakkul (trust in Allah), which, if practised during trials and tribulations, can not only increase our resilience but also strengthen our relationship with Allah. We described how sabr does not mean being passive but making changes where we can and at the times we cannot, then to have tawakkul, that despite the hardship, Allah does not burden a soul any more than it can bear.

If we go back to the story of Hajar, the wife of Ibrahim (as), remember that she did not sit passively even though she had sabr and tawakkul and was willing to endure her fate due to her faith in Allah. When her provisions ran out and her baby cried with thirst she ran between the mountains of Safa and Marwa seven times in search of water. She trusted Allah's plan but was also compelled to act herself. When she could not find any water Hajar prayed for Allah's help and in answer to her prayer, the zam zam spring burst forth from the ground. Her actions follow the principles of *"trust in Allah but also tether your camel."*

In other words, we cannot remain passive in our suffering and expect Allah to resolve our difficulties. Alongside prayer, we can practice self-management of our condition and focus on the things we can control rather than those we do not have control over.

Think of the journey of life as being guided by a compass or GPS. You may wander off track and take the wrong turn or reach a long diversion but try to keep your focus on what your values and goals are. Keep renewing your orientation to stay aligned with your values and focussed on your goals.

The Prophet ﷺ said, *"The deeds most beloved in the eyes of Allah are those deeds carried out with continuity (regularity) although they may be small"* (SahihBukhari 6465). No matter what you do remain consistent in your practice of the exercises to keep you focussed on living a values-based life as when all else ends the only thing that remains is your actions and your intentions regardless of whether you achieve success or not. *"Verily, the reward of deeds depends on the intentions, and each person will be rewarded according to what he intended"* (Sahih Bukhari 1).

For some people, chronic illness is a catastrophe that feels like their life as they knew it has ended. For others, it may be seen as a new beginning giving them a new purpose and direction even though, given the choice, they would not have wanted it to be that way. Outline the importance of using thought defusion and present-moment awareness exercises to help the client drop the struggle with thoughts and learn to sit with internal sensations and unhelpful thoughts without judgement.

No matter how hard we try, we all get caught up in the struggle with unwelcome thoughts, feelings, and sensations that we want to get rid of and do things to make them go away even when they are detrimental for us in the long term. This is because we live in a world where we are encouraged to think we can only be happy without adversities. When plans do not work out as we expect them to, we struggle with whatever life is presenting us with and create stress, anxiety, and other emotions that are difficult to manage. Yet pain and suffering are paradoxical. We hate to have pain, but without it, we are not happy because until you experience difficulty you cannot enjoy ease.

Fear is a major contributor to this process, as we are not comfortable with not knowing what lies ahead in our future. When the mind is tamed with defusion and is fully present, we can observe our thought patterns, catch the story we are creating in our minds, and establish some distance from it to avoid becoming hooked. It is then easier to focus on valued activities with better pain tolerance and eventual acceptance.

Remember to use the "Dropping Anchor" exercise which will help to bring you back to the present moment to be able to observe the storm without being caught up in it. Remind yourself constantly that life is something that happens FOR us, not TO us. Whatever experience Allah sends to us is meant to give us exactly what we need to expand. Our adversity is an opportunity to turn to Allah and to move us in the direction of spiritual growth and development.

With tawakkul, we can release the need for control, become more receptive to spiritual guidance, and begin to live a God-conscious life to drive us to meet difficult situations more effectively. The more we practice, dropping anchor, the easier it will become to drop the struggle and take committed action to align our life with our values and to move in the direction we need to move towards.

Using narratives from the Quran will serve the client as reminders that life is a matter of perspective and that increasing connection with the Quran will strengthen our relationship with Allah and help increase resilience to manage life with or without pain.

As human beings, we often feel despair in the face of trials and tribulations related to illnesses and chronic medical conditions. If thoughts such as "why me" start to creep into your mind, turning to the Quran can help us find meaning and remind us how those before us suffered trials and tribulations with faith and trust. While no one wants to suffer the tests of life, there is truth in the saying that with adversity comes strength. The Quran tells us that even Prophets were tested with pain and suffering, but, as a consolation for the human mind, there is a constant reminder that with difficulty comes ease.

While the Day of Ashura is well known for the tragic martyrdom of Imam Hussain, Islām tells us that this day was also important because relief from suffering was brought to several Prophets. On this day, Allah parted the red sea and saved Prophet Musa (AS) (Moses) from the Pharoah, the Ark of the Prophet Nuh (AS) (Noah) landed on Mount Judi saving him and his followers, Prophet Yunus (AS) (Jonah) was released from the belly of the whale, and Allah accepted the repentance of the Prophet's Adam (AS) and Dawud (AS) (David).

The last verse of sura Yusuf reminds us that the stories in the Quran were there for a purpose, as guidance and inspiration for those suffering from trials and tribulations and a consolation that they will be rewarded.

> There was certainly in their stories a lesson for those of understanding. Never was the Qur'an a narration invented, but a confirmation of what was before it and a detailed explanation of all things and guidance and mercy for a people who believe.
>
> (Quran 12:111)

Furthermore, we are told that our pain and suffering are not in vain. The Prophet Muhammed ﷺ said: *"No fatigue, disease, sorrow, sadness, harm, or distress befalls a Muslim, even if it were a prick of a thorn, but Allah will expiate some of his sins thereby"* (Sahih Bukhari 5641), meaning that no pain however insignificant is without atonement and spiritual purification. Allah promises a reward in the hereafter.

When Prophet Yusuf (AS) was thrown into the well by his jealous brothers and spent years in jail even though he was innocent of any crime, rather than harbouring anger, he used the time in prison to preach to his fellow prisoners and advance the teachings of his religion. *"My fellow prisoners, say which is better, many gods at variance, or Allah the one, the conqueror?"* (Quran 12:39). Prophet Yusuf (AS) trusted Allah to take care of him regardless of the situation he was in. With sabr and tawakkul, he rose from his misfortunes with fortitude and became a high authority in the land he was once imprisoned in. *"Certainly those who keep from evil and are patient, Allah does not let the wage of the good doers go to waste"* (Quran 12:90).

Likewise, the Quran tells us *"It may be that you dislike a thing while it is good for you, and it may be that you love a thing while it is evil for you, and Allah knows, while you do not know"* (Quran 2:216). In other words, there may be times when we experience situations that we do not want to face and cannot see the good in them at all yet there may be a bigger plan that Allah has for us that we do not yet understand.

We can take inspiration from the life of the Prophet Ayyub (AS) (Job) who even as a Prophet faced a divine test of his faith. Allah granted him immense wealth, good health, and a large family for which Prophet Ayyub (AS) constantly praised and thanked the Almighty for his blessings.

However, he became the object of severe adversity when he lost all his wealth and his children and was afflicted by an incurable and painful disease. His disease caused so much revulsion that his friends and relatives abandoned him save for his wife. Regardless, Prophet Ayyub (AS) remained patient and continued to put his trust in Allah until eventually with Allah's mercy he was cured from his disease and regained his wealth. Prophet Ayyub (AS) worshipped Allah with full submission and patience even when he was experiencing extreme distress. *"Truly! We found him patient. How excellent a slave! Verily, he was ever oft returning in repentance to Us!"* (Quran 38:44).

While the stories from the Quran are extremely powerful, it may help to provide the client with some contemporary context to shift them out of feelings of despair that as mere mortals they cannot compete with the fortitude and tawakkul shown by the Prophets.

A more contemporary example of rising from adversity is that of a client who because of his chronic pain lost his livelihood as a bricklayer which he believed was his only employable route as he had not achieved any qualifications when he left school due to undiagnosed dyslexia. The client succumbed to a state of misery and despair until a chance discussion with an employment adviser led to him being assessed and formally diagnosed with dyslexia. His diagnosis opened the doors for him to receive government funding and a laptop adapted to his needs so that he could embark on a degree course with extra support from the university to help him manage his learning disability.

As a result, the client was able to gain employment in a career that he had only dreamed of and no longer worried about being unemployable. This was his silver lining in the cloud because, if he had not suffered the injury that caused the chronic pain, he would never have pursued a different career path and would have been doomed to a life of labouring in an unfulfilling job.

Although it is hard to ever see anything good in a situation where there is pain and suffering, when we start to accept our position, we can make sense of it and may also be able to stand back and see some benefit for ourselves or others.

For example, experiencing the trauma of losing a parent may lead to the children becoming closer to Allah by establishing regular salah, praying for their parent's soul, and making supplications as a way of preventing themselves from drowning in grief. While they will always feel pain like a stab in the heart when they think of their parent's absence and wish their parent was still alive, in time they will be able to reflect on the positive changes in themselves and be grateful for the spiritual growth they have experienced because of the experience of grief and loss.

The Prophet ﷺ said,

> Wonderful is the affair of the believer, for there is good for him in every matter and this is not the case with anyone except the believer. If he is happy, then he thanks Allah and thus there is good for him, and if he is harmed, then he shows patience and thus there is good for him.
>
> (Muslim 2999)

Even if it takes years for us to see the goodness of a trial or tribulation, having trust in Allah is knowing that no matter how hard life is, there is unknown goodness in it. Hence, the importance of saying "Alhamdulillah" when good occurs and "Alhamdulillah" even when we encounter difficulty because it is a testament to our deep trust in Allah's decree. Hence, by becoming aware of the positives that may have arisen because of the difficulties each one of us faces, we can find meaning and purpose in life. We can foster our psychological and spiritual growth by simply reminding ourselves frequently of the advantages or blessings that our struggles may have brought about, even if there is only one.

As the end of the session approaches remember that some people may have the expectation that ending the sessions means being pain-free. Remind the client that chronic pain is an experience that may be with them for a long time, but they can use the contents of the treatment sessions to maximise their psychological flexibility and learn to live with pain without struggle. Refer to the handouts they have been given throughout the sessions and encourage them to continue using the material to practice and consolidate their skills. Remind them of the need to continue with their spiritual growth.

The therapeutic strategies we have covered in the sessions so far have been aimed to help you learn to live with pain optimally. Remember to integrate these into your daily life and remain consistent so that you can continue to develop psychological flexibility. Sometimes you will notice setbacks when times are more challenging, but it is during those times when it is most important to reconnect with the activities and resources you have learned, even if you do not feel like it.

As we draw to the end of the sessions, the following guidelines can be used as a maintenance plan to help you continue to build on your successes throughout this pain management journey.

Incorporate relaxation into your daily routine to recharge your mind and help reduce tension and stress in your body. Practice the body scan or progressive muscular relaxation daily incorporating the deep breathing skills you have been practising while holding on to an awareness of Allah's presence, mercy, and blessings.

People with pain often avoid exercise for fear that it will lead to flare-ups. Lack of exercise can lead to a deconditioning of the body. Exercise is beneficial as it increases blood flow, helps build muscle strength, improves immunity, and reduces inflammation, thereby reducing pain in the long term. Exercise also has a positive effect on the mind by releasing chemicals (endorphins) in the body which not only provide pain relief but also enhance mood state. Obviously, any exercise programme needs to be supervised by a specialist in chronic pain management. Speak to your GP or health specialist to refer you to a physical therapist for appropriate exercises to gradually reorient your body.

Try to build on self-efficacy gently and gradually. Some examples of increased self-efficacy whilst making sure we are not overdoing it are pacing when engaging in exercise, using a stool to sit on when cooking, breaking down domestic chores into manageable chunks, adapting the salah prayer movements according to physical ability, increasing social and family involvement steadily, and so forth. Spiritual activities such as dhikr, Quran recitation, or attending events that may have been neglected can be incrementally increased in line with other valued activities that you have previously avoided. Sometimes, it is easy to become over-optimistic and launch into an activity to get things over and done with, but this boom of activity is likely to end with you becoming debilitated the next day. Set reasonable expectations and begin by doing one-third of what you believe you are capable of. Plan the tasks that you need to do in advance and break them down into manageable segments so that you do not end up in the bust and boom cycle. If you cannot do them, that is okay. Leave them for another day, but keep the intention.

Do not lose sight of your values and goals. Remember Allah did not create us without purpose and without meaning. Keep aligned with your meaning and purpose and focus on what your values and goals are with a commitment to act upon them.

If you are taking medications for pain relief, it may be helpful to have a medication review with a prescriber to assess whether the medication is still beneficial as the prolonged use of some medications may reduce efficacy and have undesirable side effects.

Keep in mind that the central sensitization process is influenced by the way you feel, behave, and think in reaction to pain. Factors that increase the perception of pain include stress, mental health issues such as anxiety and depression, poor functional ability to engage in enjoyable activities, and over- and under-exertion. Ensure that you become aware of your triggers and use the information we have covered to mitigate any flare-ups.

Focus on the present moment while praying, while carrying out dhikr, while out walking, while washing up, while eating, and while breathing. Learn to use present-moment awareness to increase a sense of presence in front of Allah.

Practice good sleep habits and stick to the routine. Sleep is considered to be one of the signs of the greatness of Allah in Islām. A good sleep hygiene method should be followed to ensure restful sleep is achieved to help manage chronic pain and mental state.

Stay connected with family, the community, and other support systems. Having chronic pain often makes people want to avoid being with others, but it is important to allow family and friends who care about you to support you with your emotional and practical needs and to move away from avoidance behaviour towards a life aligned with your values successfully. You will need support from others to help reinforce what you are doing.

Finally, in order for you to continue with your spiritual and personal growth through the journey of managing chronic pain, remember that there is a divine wisdom behind trials and tribulations.

We will all face adversities throughout our lifetimes, some more than others. Allah puts us through both good and bad times to test the genuineness of our faith. "*It is he who created death and life to test which of you are best in deed, for he is the Almighty, the Forgiving*" (Quran 67:2). We know from the Quran and the Hadith that trials are a sign that Allah intends good for us because, through them, our sins are atoned, and are an opportunity for growth and to become closer to Allah. "*If Allah intends good for someone, then he afflicts him with trials*" (Sahih Bukhari 5645).

Maintain your communication with Allah through prayer (salah, dua dhikr, and contemplation). Spending at least 20 minutes a day in contemplative prayer and dhikr is an important spiritual practice that will activate your cognitive and spiritual faculties and increase your awareness of Allah. Dhikr in a state of presence is a form of worship that will consolidate the part of the brain that is rational with the emotional, the head with the heart, and will elevate your receptiveness for spiritual growth with tranquillity and humility.

Engage in acts of altruism. "*And they give others preference over themselves even though they were themselves in need*" (Quran 59:9). This verse was revealed in response to the amazing act of communal altruism that the Ansari tribe in Medina displayed to welcome the Muslim emigrants (muhajiroon) who were escaping from persecution from the Meccans. Their actions were so great in merit that Allah Himself praised the Ansar and promised reward in the following verse:

> *The foremost (in faith) from the Muhajiroon and the Ansar and those who follow them in righteousness; God is well-pleased with them, and they are well-pleased with Him. He has prepared for them (the Companions and their followers in righteousness) gardens under which rivers flow to dwell therein forever – that is the supreme success.*

(Quran 9:100)

Inject small acts of kindness into the routine of your daily life. Even praying for someone in need without them knowing is an act of altruism.

Remember to cultivate gratitude by appreciating small and often insignificant things to remind you of the many blessings Allah has bestowed upon you. In Surah, Rahman Allah asks us 31 times "*Which of the favours of your Lord will you deny?*" (Quran 55). This verse is a reminder to help us look for the positives in our life. Gratitude can be expressed in our hearts, through our speech and through our deeds. Even when you feel you do not have anything to be grateful for, remember that having gratitude is beneficial for you alone. "*If you are thankful, I will add more (favours) unto you but if you show ingratitude then my punishment is terrible indeed*" (Quran 14:7). It will help to use a gratitude journal to write down the things you feel grateful for every night before going to sleep.

The spiritual growth and therapeutic gains you have experienced will be maintained by the continued practice of the exercises we have discussed. One way to continue to put into practice the things you have learned is to allocate a daily routine that you devote to the worship of Allah outside of your obligatory prayer times. Set a certain time aside and use this time to read about Islām, carry out dhikr, or recite the Quran. Connect with Muslim support groups or learning circles many of which are available online which makes it easier to access a community of like-minded individuals. Use a journal to document your learning journey.

Before finishing the session, address any concerns about this session and any clarifications from the maintenance plan they might need. Reiterate the need for them to continue practising the ACT exercises to help them foster acceptance and commitment to live a valued based life with clear and practical goals. Finish the session by thanking and congratulating the client for completing the therapy programme. Provide them with Handout 2.8 (Appendix 2) to take away as their maintenance plan.

References

https://sunnah.com/muslim:2999

Sahih al-Bukhari 6465, Book 81, Hadith 54 https://sunnah.com/bukhari:6465

Sahih al-Bukhari 1, Book 1, Hadith 1

Sahih al-Bukhari 5641, 5642, Book 75, Hadith 2 https://sunnah.com/bukhari:5641

Sahih al-Bukhari 5645, Book 75, Hadith 5 https://sunnah.com/bukhari:5645

12 Conclusions

Summary

This book is an introduction to ACT and the psychological flexibility model with the aim of developing an Islāmic adaptation to be used with those living with chronic pain. The therapy described in this book is not a linear treatment plan as the processes can be delivered flexibly and interchangeably and tailored to the client's needs.

A review of the literature on the efficacy of ACT in managing chronic pain was presented, and the main components of ACT and their congruence with the tenets of Islām were described. The ACT approach to pain management was integrated with Islāmic concepts regarding pain and suffering and was delivered in a session-by-session guide to assist in the management of pain for Muslim patients. References to sources from the Quran and Hadith were used to illustrate how Islāmic concepts can be applied to the six processes of ACT.

This book is not intended to be a prescriptive manual but rather a guide to using an evidence-based treatment approach incorporating Islāmic principles for managing chronic pain. The difficulty of being trapped in the cycle of pain and stress is often related to experiential avoidance, efforts to control the uncontrollable, and the desire to eliminate the symptoms of pain. These unhelpful strategies not only exacerbate the pain experience but often lead to paralysed spiritual growth.

While the ACT model can help harness the client's inner resources to develop the psychological flexibility to use cognitive defusion, present-moment awareness, valued action, and acceptance to help them reclaim their life, the Islāmic psychotherapeutic adaptation helps redirect the client towards the rich guidance and support that Islām has given for managing pain and suffering, thereby helping them connect with the Almighty and return to the fitrah.

Chronic pain may never be eliminated, but reconnecting with Allah and His religion can help people experiencing trials and tribulations bring meaning and purpose to their life and become more reflective. The ultimate purpose is not for the client to live a pain-free and stress-free life as this can never be guaranteed but for them to live a life aligned with their values regardless of

DOI:10.4324/9781003329626-14

the situation with sabr, tawakkul, and taqwa in the knowledge that this life is a temporary abode with promises of rewards in the hereafter.

Future Directions

There is little research evidence on the use of ACT for Muslim patients experiencing chronic pain conditions. The research literature shows that both religious and spiritual beliefs influence pain management; hence, it is important to incorporate spirituality and religion in therapeutic interventions for chronic pain. Given that ACT is considered to be an effective therapy for the management of chronic pain, it is important to consider the adaptation of this model for the care of Muslim patients.

It is anticipated that the step-by-step cultural adaptation of the six core processes of ACT and the guided sessions provided in this book will enable the clinical practitioner to apply the protocol with fidelity and to be able to gather evidence-based outcome data on the effectiveness of this model. There is a strong need for an evidence base for such interventions and evaluation data that are relevant and applicable to Muslim communities. With the lack of research on Islāmic adaptations of ACT for chronic pain, future research involving larger clinical samples will shed more light on the effectiveness of using ACT with Muslim clients. This book is considered a timely endeavour to develop psychotherapy adapted to the needs of Muslims with chronic pain.

Appendices

Appendix 1

Worksheets

Worksheet 1.1 Identifying Cost Benefits of Pain Coping Strategies

Type of pain management	Short-term gains	Long term	Effect on quality of life
Taking a cocktail of painkillers daily	It eases the pain for a while	No change in pain – pain is still steady and constant	Often makes me feel drowsy and less inclined to do anything

Worksheet 1.2 Identifying Values

Instructions: The following worksheet can be used to elicit what you value and what may be preventing you from living by those values.

Step 1: Think of an activity or relationship in your life that you value, but that you have found yourself moving away from due to pain. Maybe it is a relationship you care a lot about or a spiritual activity, but you have noticed you are not as interested in it as you used to be.

Step 2: On a piece of paper. In the left box, write down what you value in that relationship or activity. How would you like to increase your valued activities?

Step 3: In the right box, write what difficult thoughts and feelings come up when you start taking action towards that value.

Value	Difficult thoughts/feelings/ behaviour
Examples: To spend more time doing activities with my children and being a good mother *To perform fajr prayers without fail*	*I feel irritable and intolerant of them because I am in pain.* *I find it hard as my body is stiff and the pain flares up.*

Worksheet 1.3 Goal Setting

Setting SMART goals.

STEP 1

Specific: Specify the actions you will take, when and where you will do so, and who or what is involved. For example, a vague or non-specific goal is: "I will make more time to recite the Quran." A specific goal is: "I will read a few pages of the Quran every day."

Meaningful: The goal should be meaningful and guided by your values, rather than following a rigid rule or trying to avoid some pain. For example, "I have neglected my religious duties and want to get back into a routine to connect with Allah so I will start by reciting the Quran regularly."

Adaptive: Is the goal likely to improve the quality of your life?

Realistic: The goal should be realistic while taking into account your health and any competing demands on your life.

Time-bound: Be specific about the goal by either setting a day or time for it for example "I will recite a few pages of the Quran every morning after fajr." If this is difficult be as specific as possible for example "I will recite a few pages of the Quran at least once a day."

Do not try to reach for a goal that is unrealistic even at the best of times. If you do, you are setting yourself up to fail. For example, setting a goal like "I will go out for a walk without feeling anxious" is a dead goal because anxiety is a feeling or state that can happen even when you do not want it to. This means that you cannot always stop it. Make sure you set goals that you can control.

STEP 2

My goals are as follows:

- Immediate goal (something small, simple, and easy, I can do in the next 24 hours)
- Short-term goals (things I can do over the next few days and weeks)
- Medium-term goal(s) (things I can do over the next few weeks and months)
- Long-term goal(s) (things I can do over the next few months and years

Adapted from Russ Harris 2008 www.thehappinesstrap.com

Worksheet 1.4 Pacing Plan

Activity	Baseline	Goal
Go for nature walks	10 minutes once a week	Increase by 5 minutes a week
Visit close family members	Once a month for an hour	To visit once a week

Appendix 2

Handouts

Handout 2:1 Deep Breathing Exercise

Instructions for deep breathing
Sit comfortably, or if you prefer, lie down. Start by noticing your breathing; pay attention to how you are breathing, and gently slow down your breathing. We are going to take deep breaths through the nose and exhale out through the mouth. The exhale will be longer and slower than the inhale. Place one hand on your abdomen and the other hand on your upper chest. Focus your breathing on your abdomen. As you breathe inhale to a count of five, and the hand on your abdomen should rise. Your abdomen should look like a balloon being inflated. Hold for three seconds and breathe out (exhale) to the count of eight, slowly through your mouth with pursed lips as though you are blowing out a candle. The abdomen should become flat against the spine like a balloon that is deflated. Your hand on your upper chest should make little movement, while the other hand should correspond with the abdomen being inflated and deflated. Take slow and gentle breaths. As you gently build this rhythm and your breathing finds a comfortable speed, focus your mind on Allah. Carry on breathing like this for about five minutes, and as you finish, take one last deep inhale, and breathe out with a long and sharp breath. Just take a moment to notice how you feel.

The key is first to master the breathing technique to calm the CNS and then to connect to the divine with dhikr. Practice this breathing technique two to three times a day for 5–10 minutes. This natural breathing technique helps reduce pain intensity and manage pain spasms and is helpful for emotional regulation at times of stress and anxiety. You will get the most benefit if you practice this regularly, as part of your daily routine.

Handout 2.2 Dropping Anchor

This exercise can be remembered by using the acronym ACE.

A: Acknowledge your thoughts and feelings
C: Come back into your body
E: Engage in what you're doing

Let us think about the pain right now and the struggle it might be creating for you.
First, acknowledge your thoughts and feelings, sensations, or urges that you may be experiencing with curiosity but without any judgement. For example, "I am noticing a thought that my pain is going to become worse" or "I am noticing some anxiety."
Second, come back into your body and connect with your physical body. You can do this by using the following strategies:
Slowly push your feet onto the floor and feel the ground beneath you; straighten your back or sit forward in your chair; slowly stretch your arms or neck and shrug your shoulders; press the tips of your fingers together.
Take a deep slow breath!
The important thing is that you do not try to avoid feelings or pain. Instead, you should stay aware of them and acknowledge that they are there. At the same time, be aware of your body as you move it.
Third, engage in what you are doing. Keep your attention on your thoughts and feelings and connect with your body by using your senses to notice five things you can see, four things you can hear, three things you can feel two things you can smell, and one thing you can taste.
By practising this regularly, it is possible to develop acceptance of the pain as it happens because you are no longer trying to fight it.

Handout 2.3 Leaves on a Stream Exercise

Leaves on a Stream Exercise

Find a comfortable position and imagine you are sitting by the side of a gently flowing stream, and leaves are floating past the surface of that stream. Once you have that image in your mind, for the next few minutes, take every thought that pops into your head, place it on a leaf, and let it float by. Do this regardless of whether your thoughts feel good or bad, pleasant, or painful. Just place them on the leaf and let them float by.
Just allow the stream to flow at its speed. If you start thinking, this is silly, or I cannot do this, place those thoughts on a leaf ("I am now thinking this is silly"). If you notice a difficult feeling arising such as impatience or frustration, simply acknowledge it. Saying to yourself, "I have a feeling of frustration" or "I notice a feeling of impatience." Then place those words on a leaf and let them float away.
From time to time, your thoughts will take over and you might lose track of the exercise. This is expected and will happen, but as soon as you realise your thoughts are beginning to wander, gently acknowledge this and then start the exercise again.

Handout 2.4 Present-Moment Awareness Exercise Using Tasbih Dhikr

Let us begin the exercise with you choosing an anchor. Focus your awareness on your breathing and start to take slow breaths just like you have learnt in the breathing exercise. You can either close your eyes or focus on a point on the floor. Scan your body and try to relax any area of your body where there may be muscle tension. With each breath, gauge the state of your heart and mind for any thoughts, feelings, or sensations, and then bring back the awareness to your breath. Take each breath with gratitude to Allah for the life and energy he has given you. Start to anchor your thoughts and roll each bead through your fingers. Be mindful of the texture of the bead while focusing on the recitation you are making. Every time your mind wanders, return your attention to Allah with an awareness of His watchful presence. Just focus on your chosen recitation while continuing to roll the tasbih beads through your fingers.

Think of your mind as if it were a still pond and your thoughts are ripples and waves in this pond. Be aware of the ripples, but remember you can also choose to ignore them as engaging in them will only make the waves stronger. Notice the waves and ripples, acknowledge them, and allow them to simply disperse while you anchor yourself and return your attention to the here and now.

Continue this practice for at least five minutes. . . .

The repeated practice will help the mind associate these recitations with the presence of the heart connected to Allah and will strengthen the ability to remain grounded in the here and now, in Allah's remembrance with the knowledge that He is always with you.

Remember that even when you are present in the moment before Allah, the mind will wander off and become distracted by emerging thoughts. Present-moment awareness in this context is not about silencing our thoughts, but simply becoming aware of them and learning to let them pass. The more conscious we are of our thoughts, the more distance we can create between ourselves and them. Only then can we stop becoming our thoughts.

With continued practice, you will strengthen your mental and spiritual ability to be able to diffuse from these thoughts and remain present in the moment. This may take time, but the more you repeat the exercise while in a state of gratitude for Allah's mercy and blessings, the easier it will become to put a distance between unhelpful thought processes and reactivity.

Handout 2.5 Practicing Gratitude

Gratitude is practised by recognising and appreciating all our blessings from the heart, reinforcing thankfulness with our tongue, and conducting righteous deeds.

To achieve the gratitude mindset, try practising the following tips daily:

1. Let the thought of Allah be your guide for the day.
2. Keep a gratitude journal and make a list of five things each day for which you are grateful.
3. Say thank you to people for the little things they do for you, for example, write a thank you note to someone who has made a positive difference in your life.
4. Consider those who are less fortunate, put yourself in their situation, feel compassion for their suffering, and take some action, no matter how tiny, to help them.
5. When challenging times arise, remember the good things in life. Things could be a lot worse!
6. Remember to smile often and remind yourself to maintain an attitude of gratitude for all the blessings you have despite having to live with pain.

Handout 2.6 Relaxation Exercise

Relaxation Exercise

Learning to relax may sound easy but it takes time and needs to be practiced every day to become an automatic response when feeling anxious. It is important to practice when you are not at your worst as otherwise it may be difficult to master and lead to loss of motivation if positive results are not immediately noticed.

To start this exercise, find a comfortable place to sit or lie down and make sure you will not be disturbed. Close your eyes and start by focusing on your breathing. Just as we have practiced deep breathing at each session get yourself comfortable and breathe deeply for a few minutes. With each out-breath release, any tension in your body and allow your limbs to become limp. Continue breathing mindfully and then start to scan your body and become aware of any sensations in your body. If you notice any discomfort or sensations, direct your attention to that part of your body and breathe into that area while allowing the sensations to happen. Pay attention to any changes of intensity to those sensations. Notice any areas of your body that have a greater intensity and describe them.

What colour is the sensation? Does it have a shape? Can you make a visual image of that sensation? Does it feel hot or cold? At the same time, continue to breathe deeply and know you are in control.

Now think about how you might change the colour, shape, and temperature of the sensation so that it feels more comfortable. Could you shrink it, soften it, or make it a lighter colour or a more calming colour? What about the temperature? Does it feel better turned up or turned down? Start with some small subtle changes to the sensation.

Continue breathing in and out while making changes to the sensations until you begin to feel the discomfort bearable and relaxed. As you start to feel more relaxed use your imagination to take your mind to a place where you feel calm, happy, and safe. It can be anywhere whether it is in the countryside, near the beach, in a place of prayer whether at home, or in a nurturing person's home. Anywhere that feels calming and relaxing. Stay there for a few minutes.

Now pay attention to your breathing again and with each breath notice that you are feeling lighter and more alert and more mindful of your surroundings and gradually return your focus to the room you are sitting in. Take four more breaths, and each time you take a breath, notice you are more alert. As you finish this exercise, open your eyes and gently stretch your body.

Sometimes, a short body scan might be preferred to induce relaxation. In this case, the following body scan can be conducted. If practiced regularly, it can be used anywhere.

Handout 2.7 Body Scan

Short Body Scan Exercise

If you notice any tension in your body or feel the stress levels rising, take a deep breath (as practised (previously) and keep breathing slowly and deeply for a few minutes. Let your shoulders droop and relax your hands. As you continue to take slow, deep breaths starting from your feet, tense and relax the muscles before moving upwards from your feet to your legs, thighs, hips, stomach, hands, arms, chest, shoulders, neck, and then your face and head. As you focus on each area of your body, tense that part, hold for a few seconds, and then let go of the tension and notice the difference.

This practice will help you become aware of what your body feels like when it is tense and how it feels when the tension is released. Try to practise it as often as possible but at least once a day if you can. Over time you will be able to do a body scan anytime, anyplace whether you are sitting down or standing, at home, or even in crowded places, and release tension from the various parts of your body.

Handout 2.8 Maintenance Plan

1. Remember to incorporate relaxation into your daily routine to recharge your body and mind and help reduce tension and stress in your body. Practice the body scan or progressive muscular relaxation daily incorporating the deep breathing skills you have been practising while holding an awareness of Allah's presence, mercy, and blessings.

2. People with pain often avoid exercise for fear that it will lead to flare-ups. Lack of exercise can lead to a deconditioning of the body. Exercise is beneficial as it increases blood flow, helps build muscle strength, improves immunity, and reduces inflammation, thereby reducing pain in the long term. Exercise also has a positive effect on the mind by releasing chemicals (endorphins) in the body which not only provide pain relief but also enhance mood state. Any exercise programme needs to be supervised by a specialist in chronic pain management. Speak to your GP or health specialist to refer you to a physical therapist for appropriate exercises to gradually reorient your body.

3. Try to build on self-efficacy gently and gradually. Some examples of increased self-efficacy whilst making sure we are not overdoing it are pacing when engaging in exercise, using a stool to sit on when cooking, breaking down domestic chores into manageable chunks, adapting the salah prayer movements according to physical ability, increasing social and family involvement steadily, and so forth. Spiritual activities such as dhikr, Quran recitation, or attending events that may have been neglected can be incrementally increased in line with other valued activities that you have previously avoided.

4. Avoid boom and bust as it is likely to end with you becoming debilitated the next day. Set reasonable expectations and begin by doing one-third of what you believe you are capable of. Plan the tasks that you need to do in advance and break them down into manageable segments so that you do not end up in the bust and boom cycle. If you cannot do them, that is okay. Leave them for another day, but keep the intention.

5. Do not lose sight of your values and goals. Remember Allah did not create us without purpose and meaning. Keep aligned with your meaning and purpose and focus on what your values and goals are with a commitment to act upon them.

6. If you are taking medications for pain relief, it may be helpful to have a medication review with a prescriber to assess whether the medication is still beneficial as the prolonged use of some medications may reduce efficacy and have undesirable side effects.

Handout 2.8 (Continued)

7. Keep in mind that the central sensitization process is influenced by the way you feel, behave, and think in reaction to pain. Factors that increase the perception of pain include stress, mental health issues such as anxiety and depression, poor functional ability to engage in enjoyable activities, and over- and under-exertion. Ensure that you become aware of your triggers and use the information we have covered to mitigate any flare-ups.

8. Present-moment awareness practice does not have to be complicated. Focus on the present moment while praying, while conducting dhikr, while out walking, while washing up, while eating, and while breathing. Learn to use present-moment awareness to increase a sense of presence in front of Allah.

9. Practice good sleep habits and stick to the routine. Sleep is considered to be one of the signs of the greatness of Allah in Islām. A good sleep hygiene method should be followed to ensure restful sleep is achieved to help manage chronic pain and mental state.

10. Stay connected with family, the community, and other support systems. Having chronic pain often makes people want to avoid being with others, but it is important to allow family and friends who care about you to support you with your emotional and practical needs and to move away from avoidance behaviour towards a life aligned with your values successfully. You will need support from others to help reinforce what you are doing.

11. Maintain your communication with Allah through prayer (salah, dua dhikr, and contemplation). Spending at least 20 minutes a day in contemplative prayer and dhikr is an important spiritual practice that will activate your cognitive and spiritual faculties and increase your awareness of Allah. Dhikr in a state of presence is a form of worship that will consolidate the part of the brain that is rational with the emotional, the head with the heart, and will elevate your receptiveness for spiritual growth with tranquillity and humility.

12. Engage in acts of altruism. "And they give others preference over themselves even though they were themselves in need" (Quran 59:9). Inject small acts of kindness into the routine of your daily life. Even praying for someone in need without them knowing is an act of altruism.

13. Remember to cultivate gratitude by appreciating small and often insignificant things to remind you of the many blessings Allah has bestowed upon you. A gratitude journal can help with this, where you can jot down the things you feel grateful for every night before going to sleep.

Index

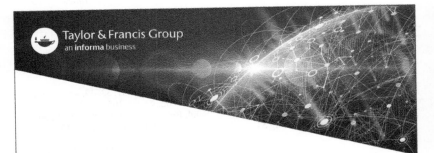

For Product Safety Concerns and Information please contact our EU
representative GPSR@taylorandfrancis.com Taylor & Francis Verlag GmbH,
Kaufingerstraße 24, 80331 München, Germany

Printed and bound by CPI Group (UK) Ltd, Croydon, CR0 4YY
08/06/2025
01896998-0009